Doctors' Dilemmas

Doctors' Dilemmas

Moral Conflict and Medical Care

SAMUEL GOROVITZ

OXFORD UNIVERSITY PRESS

New York   Oxford

Oxford University Press

Oxford   New York   Toronto
Delhi   Bombay   Calcutta   Madras   Karachi
Kuala Lumpur   Singapore   Hong Kong   Tokyo
Nairobi   Dar es Salaam   Cape Town
Melbourne   Auckland

and associated companies in
Beirut   Berlin   Ibadan   Mexico City   Nicosia

First published in 1982 by Macmillan Publishing Co., Inc., New York
First issued in paperback in 1985 by Oxford University Press, Inc.,
200 Madison Avenue, New York, NY 10016
Reprinted by arrangement with the author

Library of Congress Cataloging in Publication Data
Gorovitz, Samuel.
Doctors' dilemmas.
Reprint. Originally published: New York : Macmillan, c1982.
Bibliography: p.
Includes index.
1. Medical ethics.   I. Title.   [DNLM: 1. Ethics, Medical.
2. Philosophy, Medical. W 50 G672d   1982a]
R724.G68   1985   174'.2   85-10525
ISBN 0-19-503695-6 (pbk.)

The author gratefully acknowledges permission to reprint from
Cancer Ward by Alexander Solzhenitsyn. English translation © The Bodley Head Ltd., 1968. Reprinted by permission of Farrar, Straus & Giroux, Inc., New York.
"How Virtues Become Vices: Medicine and Social Context" by Alasdair MacIntyre in *Evaluation
and Explanation in the Biomedical Sciences: Proceedings of the First Trans-disciplinary Sym-
posium on Philosophy and Medicine* edited by H. Tristram Englehardt, Jr., and Stuart F. Spicker.
Copyright © 1975 by D. Reidel Publishing Company, Dordrecht, Holland. Reprinted by permission of the publisher.
Oblomov by Ivan Goncharov, translated by Ann Dunnigan. Copyright © 1963 by Ann Dunnigan.
Reprinted by arrangement with The New American Library, Inc., New York.
Patient Care Techniques by Dorothy J. Hicks. Copyright © 1975 by Bobbs-Merrill. Reprinted by
permission of Bobbs-Merrill, Indianapolis, Ind.
Whose Life Is It Anyway? by Brian Clark. Reprinted by permission of Mr. Clark. For information
on amateur performance rights in the U.S., contact The Dramatic Publishing Co., 4150 North
Milwaukee Ave., Chicago, Illinois 60641. For stock performance, contact Samuel French, 25
W. 45th St., New York, New York 10036. In the United Kingdom contact Amber Lane Press,
The Slack, Ashover, Derbyshire S45 OEB.

Printing (last digit): 9 8 7 6 5 4 3 2 1

Printed in the United States of America

For Judie

Contents

Preface to the Paperback Edition

MANY NEW ISSUES in medical ethics have arisen since this book first appeared. Baby Fae had a baboon heart implanted, several men had artificial hearts installed, advertisements for surrogate mothers have offered payments of $50,000, the Baby Doe Hotline saga ran its course, review procedures for genetic therapy are in place, there has been a massive movement into health care of for-profit corporations, fetal surgery has increased, embryo freezing and transfer have taken place, proposals to establish commercial markets in kidneys have been debated and defeated, and more. Many topics of current concern are thus not addressed in this book. But many topics were left out at the time it was written, as well. For the book was never meant to be exhaustive; its point was to illustrate modes of thought by addressing selected issues. The expanding agenda of problems in medical ethics only increases the need for understanding those modes of thought that can be used to address them constructively.

Not much would change if I were rewriting the book today. I still maintain the guarded optimism, for which I argue here at length, about our collective ability to forge solutions to most of the problems we confront in medical ethics. I would, however, place considerably greater emphasis on two points.

First, I would be more explicit in characterizing the value of personal autonomy, staunchly defended in the text. Autonomy is valuable in order that we may pursue our aspirations and express our distinctive characters; that much is clear to everyone. I would take greater pains to emphasize that our aspirations are fundamentally interpersonal, as is our character as individuals. The point is not merely that we do not live in isolation—that the lives we lead as individuals are intertwined with the lives of others. It goes deeper; what and who we are is itself a product of our connectedness with our backgrounds and with others in our environment. Our structures of knowledge, our characters and personalities, our language and the formation of the concepts in terms of which our aspirations are cast are all inherently social. In this context autonomy is advocated as a value, and in that advocacy there is no denial of the fundamentally social nature of moral choice. Since ethics is a social construct for the enhancement of relations among people, the social dimensions of moral challenge are always of central significance.

Second, I would assert much more strongly that physicians and patients have demonstrably different perceptions of the intimate interactions that bind them together. This book is in part a plea for, and an attempt to contribute to, a greater degree of mutual understanding between health care providers and patients. I now see more clearly the diversity and the depth of the mutual misperceptions in medical care, and therefore the need for increased candor and improved communication. But that is another story.

I am indebted to Patricia Williams for her persistence in urging that this book be made more widely available in paperback. It has been a pleasure to work with Marjorie Mueller, William Sisler, and Ellen Chodosh of Oxford University Press; they have my gratitude for making this edition a reality.

S.G.

Preface

THIS BOOK is about ethical problems in medicine and how philosophy can help us all deal with them. These problems—how physicians and patients should interact, how to deal with illness and death, how to allocate scarce medical resources, and how to decide what to believe about issues like abortion, medical errors, and sensitive questions about reproduction—affect us all, doctor and patient, nurse and family member, taxpayer and health planner, student and professional. I thus address these remarks to all such readers, presupposing only that they share an interest in exploring the subject matter.

Some colleagues have urged me to aim at a more clearly specified readership—medical students or the nonprofessional public or patients or health planners, suggesting, for example, that I decide between those who will read from the physician's point of view and those who have the patient's perspective. But why should these perspectives be so separate as to require different modes of writing? Perhaps part of what limits the success of contemporary medical practice is precisely the lack of shared viewpoint and common experience. And why should readers be compartmentalized according to the roles they happen to play at a particular moment? Physicians become patients from time to time; nurses, like other citizens, are subject to national health policies; health planners become family members of the dying. So we are all in this together. Insofar as people filling different roles have a shared perspective on matters of medical care, there is no reason why they should not read the same books. Insofar as their perspectives differ because of their different roles, they may profit from the contemplation of perspectives other than their own.

Because the physician is typically the central actor in the dramas of clinical medicine, and because clinical medicine typically provides the setting in which the issues that concern me here arise, I will pay particular attention to questions about the behavior of physicians. I want to explore what is involved in being and in becoming a good doctor, not merely in the sense of technical competence but in the sense of moral goodness. But I am also concerned with the work of another kind of doctor, the doctor of philosophy whose special interest is a greater understanding of what moral goodness is.

Doctors of the first kind—of medicine—are concerned with the treatment of illness and injury. In the course of clinical practice they are expected to act effectively and to act rightly. To varying degrees, some of them succeed and some of them fail. The challenge to act rightly, especially in the face of the increasingly difficult ethical dilemmas that beset clinical practice, demands courage and moral sensitivity. Doctors of the second kind—moral philosophers—are concerned with achieving a deeper understanding of moral values, moral conflict, and the prospects for finding solutions to moral dilemmas. They are concerned with the study of rightness itself. One question that shapes this book is whether doctors of the first kind, and their patients, colleagues, and neighbors, stand to learn anything useful from doctors of the second kind; whether those who face the realities of ethical conflict in clinical practice or in the setting of health policy can benefit, in their efforts to act rightly, from the insights and arguments of those for whom moral judgment itself is the object of interest.

I believe that clinical medicine and the setting of health policy do stand to benefit from a consideration of what moral philosophy has to say about medicine. My defense of this belief does not appear within this book; rather, it is the book as a whole that I offer in evidence. Because I am construing medicine in the broadest sense—including not just the way physicians and patients interact but the way social decisions about medical issues are made—the focus will shift from chapter to chapter, ranging over such diverse issues as what constitutes a good patient, how federal policy should be determined in ethically controversial areas, and how changes in medical education can increase the likelihood that doctors of medicine will be good doctors. The theme that unifies this diverse menu of topics is the conviction that all of these issues are properly of widespread public concern, and all of them can be helpfully illuminated by philosophical consideration.

This book is not a comprehensive treatise. It is not a survey of the philosophically challenging issues in medicine or a systematic textbook. Rather, it is a personal exploration, intended to provide a provocative introduction to a sampling of important problems and to infectious modes of thought that can entice the reader on to deeper and more definitive thought. It is not a scholarly book, laden with footnotes and uncompromising in rigor of argument. I accept some highly plausible claims as plausible enough to rely on without proof, I accept various philosophical positions without defending them, and I affirm certain propositions about medicine and health without elaborate support (though I refer the reader to documentation where I think that might be helpful). The result is a work of applied philosophy, not one that treats questions at the foundations of philosophical thought. My objectives are to offer a book that is accessible to the nonprofessional general reader; to reveal some of the character, vitality, and value of a philosophical approach—both its method and its substance—and to illuminate some aspects of medical practice, health policy, and medical education that are important not only to health care providers but to the public.

Why should the reader persevere through the pages of this book? It depends to some extent on who the reader is. One should not expect to find, within these pages, comprehensive answers to moral problems that arise in clinical medicine or health policy. But some readers may discern, here and there, the outlines of a congenial solution to one problem or another. And the general response, I hope, will be at least to put the volume down with a lingering concern about some new questions and a lasting sense of some new ways to think about them.

Medical practice intensifies our awareness of our aspirations, our frailty, our limitations, and our achievements. It touches every dimension of life. Philosophy is traditionally and properly concerned with such large issues, and medicine and health policy are thus natural subjects for philosophical reflection. My objective here is to illustrate and advocate such reflection, not to determine where it will lead.

Acknowledgments

IT HAS BEEN my extremely good fortune over the last several years to have had numerous opportunities to discuss ethical problems in medicine and health care with a broad range of people including practicing physicians, patients, medical school faculty and students, nurses, hospital administrators, government health officials at state and federal levels, educators in nursing, pharmacy and public health, and others as well. I have also had the immense benefit of association with my professional colleagues in and around philosophy. Such merit as this book may have is due largely to the insights and generosity of all these people. For example, much of what I say is illustrated with accounts of real cases—information I never would have gained but for the readiness of others to share their experiences with me. As I reflect on the extent to which my views have been shaped by these conversations, I realize the impossibility of acknowledging adequately the debts that I owe. I must therefore restrict my expressions of gratitude to those who have played a direct role in helping to make this manuscript better than it otherwise would have been. And they are many.

David and Anne Pears and Derek Parfit, by making me welcome at Oxford University in 1980, helped me produce a first draft. I was then able to learn much about its defects from the participants in my seminar for health care educators, sponsored by the National Endowment for the Humanities. They were Will Albrink, Patricia Baker, Marilyn Birchfield, Ann Marie Brooks, Donald Char, I. Bruce Gordon, Edmund Howe, Armand Karow, Ronica Kluge, Betty Mawardi, Arthur Sanders, Sumer Verma, and Floyd Westendorp. I was also helped by the reactions of an honors program faculty discussion group at the University of Maryland, composed of Margaret Bridwell, Faith Gabelnick, Jean Grambs, John

Howarth, Gary Pavela, Joan Segal, Mady Segal, Bob Shoenberg, John Splaine, Pam Splaine, and Matt Whalen.

Several other individuals read all or part of the manuscript at one stage or another and provided comments that made a significant difference: Margaret Pabst Battin, Susan Blumenthal, Arthur Caplan, Michael Eliastam, Dorothy Henneman, Larry McCullough, Douglas MacLean, Ruth Macklin, Norman Weissman, and Daniel Wikler. And Edmund Howe merits an extra mention for arranging for a draft to be read by an entire class at the Uniformed Services University of the Health Sciences. All of these people have my gratitude for their interest, encouragement, and suggestions.

At various times I have had support for work on other projects which have played a role in the development of the views contained here; I therefore acknowledge with thanks the support I have had from the National Endowment for the Humanities, the Rockefeller Brothers Fund, and the National Center for Health Services Research.

Portions of the chapter on medical mistakes are derived from "Toward a Theory of Medical Fallibility," coauthored with Alasdair MacIntyre. I appreciate his willingness to let me include that material here; what is of value in it is equally his, but he is wholly innocent of its faults.

All that help notwithstanding, the project would have come to naught but for the valiant efforts of Frances DiCarlo, Sheila Morgan, and Susan Ragland, who typed tenaciously while confronting the mysteries of a new word processor.

Joan Callahan deserves special mention for her wise and able contributions as a research assistant. And Jane Cullen, my editor at Macmillan, has been all one could reasonably hope for in an editor, providing enthusiasm, sound advice, and unfailing good humor.

At times, I feared that my account of what is involved in being a good doctor set too high a standard; remembering that Robert A. Fischer meets that standard emboldened me to hold firm.

Finally, I'm most grateful to Judie, Heidi, and Eric Gorovitz, for infusing the whole undertaking with their unwavering love.

PART ONE

Overviews

1
Moral Mayhem in Modern Medicine

I WANT TO CONSIDER medicine afresh, as if it were wholly unfamiliar. The fact, of course, is that we all are bombarded with perceptions of the world of clinical practice; they come to us through the news media, through conversations with others, through our own experiences as patients, and through various forms of entertainment that include medical themes. Further, these perceptions are colored by attitudes and beliefs about illness and physicians that are widely shared throughout our culture. Widely held beliefs and attitudes can nonetheless be bizarre to those who do not share them, and we may stand to learn something about an enterprise such as medicine by pretending to be free of those beliefs and attitudes that constitute the prevailing cultural understanding of it.

Obvious truths are often the hardest to defend. I can easily deal with someone who denies that magnesium burns brightly; I show him a chemistry text or go to a laboratory and let him see for himself. It is harder to demonstrate the difference between dreaming and being awake. Any experience you can have is one you can also dream that you are having; therefore, it seems impossible ever to be sure that you are awake, no matter what you are experiencing, and not asleep, dreaming that you are having those experiences. Pinching, the traditional nostrum for uncertainty about one's state, obviously won't work since one can dream that one is pinched and then awakens from a dream. So, as you read this page, you may not be awake at all! You may be asleep, dreaming that you are reading a philosophy book about medicine. How can you prove that you are really awake?

This sort of puzzle led the seventeenth-century French philosopher René Descartes to devise an elaborate theory of how knowledge is possible.[1] A theory of knowledge—an epistemology—is a complicated bit of business at best, far less likely to be persuasive than the simple propositions it is developed to explain or justify—propositions like the claim that you are now awake and reading, rather than asleep and dreaming. You *are* awake, and that is obvious to you, but *proving* the truth of that obvious claim is difficult—if, indeed, it is possible at all. Yet the attempt to find such a proof can lead into sophisticated areas of philosophical inquiry and hence to great insight into the nature and possibility of knowledge.

Some claims about medicine and health seem as obviously true as the claim that you are awake, and, like that claim, may be hard to defend. One such claim is that curing or preventing illness is always good to do. Another is that it is good to save lives. These claims are part of the fabric of our understanding of medicine; they seem to need no defense or justification. Nor is it clear how they could be defended if we were to make the attempt. Yet an examination of these claims can help us understand what medicine is about and how it sometimes goes wrong. Further, when we reflect on how we might be able to defend certain claims that seem to need no defense, we sometimes discover to our surprise that we may not be dealing with truths at all.

Let us consider what medicine might look like to one who knows nothing about it. The exercise should not be difficult. Imagine a distant planet on which life is like that on Earth, with one major exception. There is no illness or injury; people live to a standard age of, say, ninety years, and then, quite predictably, they instantaneously die. There are lawyers to write wills and morticians to handle funerals, but the role of the physician is unknown. Now imagine a visitor from such a place asking one of our physicians what he or she does. "I'm a doctor of medicine," replies the physician. The answer does not help, for our visitor does not understand. "I treat sick people, cure illness, save lives," explains the physician to no avail. At this point the baffled visitor might well propose an empirical solution. "Don't try to explain any more; just let me follow you around for a while and observe what you do. That way I'll be able to see for myself what the practice of medicine is."

A good political cartoon is obviously a satire, yet it captures a truth or insight. The following account should be understood in the spirit of such cartoons. For the visitor might well see the following events. The physician approaches a virtual stranger in a small, austere room. The stranger, who has been waiting a long time, looks up anxiously, yet with some relief, as the physician enters. Calling the stranger by a first name, the physician introduces himself as Dr. Whatever and directs the stranger to remove his clothes. The events that then ensue, perhaps over many days, strike our observer as barely credible; the physician examines the exterior of the stranger and then begins to examine the interior, placing instruments of various kinds in all the existing orifices and from time to time creating new orifices for the purpose. The physician directs the stranger to eat certain poisonous chemicals. The stranger complies, but his cooperation seems to do him little good. The physician perseveres, causing to be connected to the victim tubes through which additional chemicals are inserted. At one point the victim is stabbed with a sharp weapon, through which poison is inserted into the body, rendering him unconscious. The physician's henchmen then seize the fallen victim and cart him off to a room filled with various instruments—the visitor is reminded here of the Tower of London—and the punishment then escalates. The physician cuts the victim open and looks over the interior parts. He steals one or more of them, discarding them or sending them away, and sews what is left of the victim back together. Only many days later is the victim—perhaps one should say "prisoner"—let out on parole.

We could not blame the observer for concluding that the practice of medicine is a part of the penal system—indeed, the part that metes out the most severe punishments and humiliations to the worst among Earthly criminal elements. He might then observe that on his planet there are also criminals from time to time, but that the kind of invasive physical and psychological abuse he has just witnessed has long since been rejected by the judicial system as not befitting a humane and civilized social order.

"No, no," our physician protests. "It isn't punishment. This has nothing to do with the penal system. These are not prisoners or criminals."

And the visitor replies, "Then what you people call the practice of medicine I would describe as felonious assault."

Of course, this little story rests entirely on the assumption that the visitor does not understand what he is seeing; he does not know that the actions performed by the physician are designed to benefit the patient. Indeed, he does not understand the notion of being a patient. He simply observes behavior and makes of it what he can. Since *we* know what is going on, the story strikes us as ludicrous (except where it strikes a familiar chord). Yet it makes a point, for physicians do things that *would* be felonious assault except under very special circumstances of justification. And of course, the story also rests on the particular episodes the visitor chanced to see. He might well have witnessed scenes of obvious kindness instead. Still, we can understand the observer's reaction; we can sense how cruel and primitive medical practice could look to one who came to it with no prior understanding of its purpose or justification.

This fact—that much of what is done in the course of medical practice looks rather like assault—is the first of several clues that there is something quite puzzling about medicine. I do not mean, of course, merely that medicine would be puzzling to one who does not understand it; rather, I mean that medicine is a genuinely puzzling enterprise. We will understand better just how puzzling it is if we consider the various clues that we can uncover when we overcome, even partially, our customary familiarity with medical practice.

A recent joke provides another clue. A man was dying in a modern hospital. His condition was hopeless, his pain severe, his deterioration inexorable. But with pumps and pipes, tricks and tubes, the physicians kept him alive for several weeks before the end finally came. As his soul rose toward his final reward, he thought it a blessing to be free at last from the burdens of corporeal existence, free from illness and suffering, and free from the relentless beneficence of the healing arts. As he was checking in at the heavenly front desk, however, he was horrified to see someone rush by in a white coat, with a stethoscope hanging out of one pocket, carrying a black bag, with a look of great importance and urgency. The new arrival expressed his dismay to the concierge: "Pete, I am shattered. I thought that here, finally, there would be no illness and no need for medicine."

"Oh, don't let that bother you," replied Saint Peter. "That's just God playing doctor."

The possibility of such a joke rests on the familiarity of the expression *playing God* as used to describe what physicians often do. The joke can be told because its punch line reverses a well-known phrase. Substitute any other profession in the joke, and it is destroyed. Why is the notion of playing God so closely linked with the practice of medicine? And why is it that if there is one social role to which God might plausibly be imagined to aspire, it is that of the physician? Even among those occupations that enjoy wealth or vital powers—such as tycoons, generals, or Supreme Court justices—there is something special about the role of physician that makes it, uniquely, the profession that is viewed as pretending to divinity. Let this be clue number two.

And who among us has not heard the expression *doctor's orders*? Is the familiarity of that expression a result of the importance to us of abiding by the special expertise of our physicians, lest we come to grief? We also need the help of lawyers from time to time and risk losing property, freedom, or opportunities without it. Yet one does not typically hear of lawyer's orders; rather, it is legal advice that we get from members of the bar. Why this air of militaristic hierarchy in the practice of medicine? Clue number three.

The fourth clue concerns the powerful effect that the manipulation of names and titles can have on interpersonal relationships. For example, I knew a professor in graduate school who disliked one student—call him Waffle. The professor—call him Waver—dealt with most students, reciprocally, on a first-name basis. But Waver's treatment of the disliked student was diabolical. Whenever that student addressed him as Professor Waver, he responded casually, using Waffle's first name. This led Waffle to join the others in calling Waver by *his* first name. But then Waver became formal, calling the student *Mr.* Waffle. I'm not sure that Waffle ever understood; mainly, he seemed always off-balance around Waver, never knowing quite what was wrong.

I write these words in Oxford, England, mindful of the heavy weight of English history on contemporary British society. Earls and Dukes, Marquesses and Barons, and Sirs and Lords of every sort are much in evidence still, as is what seems to an American to be a hardy strain of class stratification. If one looks at the founding documents of American democracy, one finds that we, in contrast, are by quite deliberate design a nation without a titled aristocracy. No House of Lords for us, nor peerages to covet. Yet some among us do bear titles. The military is full of them, as are most institutions organized on a military model, such as rescue squads or the Boy Scouts. And some professionals mark their own with honorific labels, such as those enjoyed by the uncharitable Professor Waver. Reflect for a moment on how some of these titles work.

At a typical American university the professors hold doctoral degrees. It is therefore appropriate to address them as Professor This or Dr. That. But it is hardly expected. Especially if the university is one of substantial stature, it will suffice to address the faculty as Miss or as Mr. If a student says, "Ms. Didact, I'd like to speak with you after class," when Ms. Didact could have been addressed as Dr. or as Professor, it won't likely even be noticed. And clergymen have titles, too. If a member of the congregation says, "Mr. Vicarspiel, I'd like to speak with you after the sermon," instead of addressing him as Reverend Vicarspiel, the difference may be noticed but will be forgiven. But call a physician in clinical practice Mr. or Ms., and you learn what indignation can be. If the physician is above reacting directly, the palace guard of ancillary personnel can be relied upon to make it clear that you simply *do not* address Doctor that way.

If this seems an overstatement, I propose a simple experiment. I have done it enough to be confident of the result. Find a group containing mostly physicians, and ask them to perform this one simple task: to take a slip of paper and write on it their names; nothing more, just their names. That is a task almost any person over the age of about six can perform. But medical people seem to suffer from an occupational ailment; a large number of them cannot do it! Instead, they write something more elaborate, like "Julia Jones, M.D." Earning an M.D. degree is a considerable achievement, and taking some measure of pride in it is easily understandable. But it is, after all, simply part of one's educational history. The Ph.D. in philosophy also takes a bit of doing, but no philosopher would ever think that his *name* included Ph.D. What is there about the medical profession that leads its practitioners to think that earning a medical degree constitutes such a fundamental transformation in their very essence that it can properly be marked only by a change in the name itself? This special, intense need that physicians have to be labeled as doctors is our fourth clue that medicine is a puzzling trade.

I will cite one last clue. Just as names and titles reflect currents of power and influence in a social community, so does the manipulation of time. Perhaps the most widespread and laughable example is the bureaucratic game of who gets on the line first. You wait for your superiors to pick up the telephone when they are ready for you. Your recompense is that your subordinates wait until you are ready for them. Power is being waited for; lesser importance is waiting.

Patients wait for physicians.[2] They wait with amazing complacency, given the frequent incivility of it. Physicians *do* have severe demands on their time, and they *do* often have good reasons for being behind schedule. But often they are so insensitive that they do not even participate in the minimal conventions of common courtesy. If I am late for an appointment with a student, I believe the student is entitled to as accurate as possible a prediction of when I will be available and an apology for the delay. This is nothing more than respect for the person who awaits me— acknowledgment that his or her time is also of value and is wasted only at some loss. There is nothing unusual about this attitude; most practitioners in most professions seem to share it. The glaring exception is medicine, in which the patient is expected to be patient (this is no linguistic coincidence) and uncomplaining and may see the physician only after a very considerable wait—sometimes half an hour or more—without so much as a word of regret being expressed for the delay.

I am convinced that this rudeness is quite unintended on the part of most physicians. Rather, it is so much a part of the conventions of practice to which they are bred in the process called professionalization that they are unable to see it for what it is. Sometimes, when it is pointed out, they see the point at once, with apparent surprise that something so obvious could have escaped their attention for so long.

A radiológist once kept a member of my family waiting for ninety minutes before breezing in and setting to work, without a word about the delay. Later I had him paged at his hospital and asked him to explain this appalling behavior. He was almost speechless with shock; in more than a decade of practice no one had ever complained before about being kept waiting! Yet he readily admitted to irritation when *he* was kept waiting for an appointment and granted at once that in any other setting— such as showing up ninety minutes late for a social engagement—he would be well armed with explanations and apologies. An outpouring of apologies and affirmations of reform then followed, but I have no evidence about whether this resulted in a subsequent change of behavior.

Physicians are not always so receptive to complaint, however. I can perhaps best illustrate with an example that requires a word of introduction. I have been intrigued that an earlier draft of this chapter has been criticized as being too kind to physicians and as being too critical of physicians. The first criticism comes mainly from nonphysicians, especially those with substantial experience as patients. The second criticism comes mainly from medical students, who have an idealized image of the profession to which they aspire. On one occasion a dozen people, mainly nonphysicians, gathered to discuss that earlier draft, and the dialogue that follows is a verbatim transcript of a portion of their conversation (with names changed). I call it "Ann's Lament."

ANN: I just had an accident, and I am going to an absolutely dismal person.

BILL: An absolutely what?

ANN: Dismal. He's just terrible. I hate him.

BILL: Doctor?

ANN: Doctor. He said, "Are you doing your exercises? Are you applying heat? You're a *good* patient."

CARLA: A pat on the head; "you're a cute little thing"?

ANN: Yes, and I heard him down the hall talking to another person who was a younger person who was questioning him: "Do you realize I'm a *doctor*? Do you realize that I know what I am doing? How *dare* you question me? Who do you think you are?" I could hear this all the way down the hall.

DON: I guess I've got to ask: Why the hell are you going to this guy?

ANN: I am going to him because he is the fourth orthopedic surgeon I have been

to in a year for a variety of reasons. They are uniformly idiots and awful
people. And if I could find another one, I would go, but I am just gritting
my teeth and going.

BILL: And he has a reputation as a good technician?

ANN: And he has a reputation as being a good technician. But as a person,
forget it.

DON: Of course, I'd have to say I can't separate the two.

ANN: Well, I have to.

CARLA: Have you said anything to him?

ANN: Oh, yes.

DON: There is a morality involved in this, and there is a technical point of view
involved in this, and you've got to have both; otherwise, you're going to
be a lousy doctor. Not to mention a lousy person.

ANN: I don't agree. They are getting away with it. This guy is getting away
with it. This guy made me wait an hour and a half. When he came in, I
said, "I just waited an hour and a half!" He said, "So what?" I said, "So
what? My time is worth a lot of money." He said, "Well, you can just
walk right out of here. You're the one who came." He's right, you know.

BILL: She went to four losers, and she is assuming that if she kept going and
running into doctors—

ANN: Who has time for that?

BILL: —that they would all be losers.

ED: If you go to four supermarkets and they all have lousy tomatoes, you figure
out that they are not going to be any good anyplace.

So physicians often act in assaultive ways, are widely viewed by others
as having pretensions to divinity, package their advice in the trappings
of orders, guard their titles with a jealousy suggestive of deposed aristocracy, and often are systematically rude to their patients. Yet they are
accorded places of honor in the social order, are allowed almost unconstrained freedom to do as they see fit, and are rewarded with incomes
that would make the average professor's head spin. Surely this is puzzling
and stands in need of explanation. There must be more to the story than
I have told.

We have glimpsed the dark side of medical practice, but there is plainly
another side as well. Physicians flourish because they provide a service
that we want. They offer us expertise with respect to our health—they
help us prevent, live with, or cure our illnesses and injuries, and they
help us sustain our lives. Of course, they don't do so with complete
success; there is error in medical practice, and physicians do a substantial
amount of harm in their efforts to serve their patients. But on balance
we think of them as doing good in an important way, and that accounts

for the fact that medicine as an activity continues to exist. But it does not account for our acceptance of the phenomena I have described above.

Part of what underlies these phenomena is that we all are potential patients. Every one of us at some level, some dimly and some quite explicitly, is aware of the frailty of health and, indeed, of the fragility of life itself. Health and life can end for us or for our loved ones at a moment's notice or with no notice at all. This is a humbling and frightening realization. And it is precisely with respect to health and life—and the tragic phenomena of suffering and death—that physicians are understood to have special expertise and special powers, powers of intervention which we hope will be used benevolently in our interests, but which we fear can be withheld to our detriment or can even injure us. That fear is not irrational, given the harm that physicians sometimes do, despite the fact that on balance—at least in recent years—they do more good than harm. The harm they do is not primarily because of shabby medical practice, although there is a lot of that about. Rather, it is mainly because medical practice is necessarily in part a guessing game, and hence medicine is exceedingly difficult to do well. (One Public Health Service official has estimated that one hospital day in seven results from iatrogenic—that is, physician-caused—illness or injury.) So becoming a patient is high-risk behavior, but not becoming one is sometimes even higher-risk behavior. We therefore enter into relationships with physicians because we want something from them: a betterment of our circumstances, which can be purchased only at certain substantial costs.

If you recall now that the physician's expertise concerns our health and our life itself and that the physician has special training and special powers with respect to these goods, it is no wonder there is a tendency to revere doctors' orders. For even the physician who couches his opinions in the gentlest form of suggestion speaks against the backdrop of our awareness of his awesome power and our shattering fragility. Disobey your doctor's orders, then, at your peril. And what precisely is the risk that you then run? Not inconvenience or loss of property but, in the extreme case, capital punishment! That is the threat implicit in every medical recommendation, so the pronouncements of the physician induce a disposition to acquiesce on the part of the patient. It is no wonder that we tend to be meek in the face of medical rudeness and deferential in the face of medical arrogance.

If the physician's orders are compelling, it is important that the scope over which the physician has jurisdiction be a scope with respect to which the physician really does have legitimate authority and the appropriate expertise. Imagine this fictional transaction: Your physician says, "I want you to take methyl prednisolone acetate, to give up smoking, to stop eating crustaceans, to get more exercise, to abandon your lover, to vote Republican, and to trade your Volvo in on an Oldsmobile." Somewhere along that spectrum you get the feeling that the transaction has gone awry. With respect to the methyl prednisolone acetate, you are likely willing to go along. The advice about smoking and exercise plainly makes good medical sense, and you will likely view the advice as legitimate even if you do not follow it. With respect to the crustaceans, you think there must be some physiological situation which makes that an appropriate prohibition, and you might well inquire about that. (Of course, if it comes to light that your physician is a member of a small cult of physicians who worship the crab, then you resist his suggestion as somehow transcending the scope of legitimate medical authority.) But when you are told to stop running around with Mary-Sue, voting Democratic, and driving a Volvo, you're entitled to say, "You've crossed the border from what is your business to what is not your business."

What is the physician's proper business then? Your health; not your politics, not your romantic affiliations, not your investments—just your health. But what is that? If the physician can give orders with respect to health, but not otherwise, it is important to know what health is. The World Health Organization of the United Nations has something to say about this matter; the preamble to its constitution provides a definition: "Health is a state of complete physical, mental, and social well-being and not merely the absence of disease or infirmity."[3] If this is an acceptable definition of health, think of the consequence when the physician is considered an expert with respect to health. A visit to the physician might go like this:

PATIENT: Doctor, I'm glad to see you. I'm not well.
DOCTOR: What seems to be the trouble?
PATIENT: My social well-being is really poor. I haven't been out on a date in months. I'm lonely.
DOCTOR: I think we can do something about that. I'm writing you a prescription for a very effective computer dating service. And I'm prescribing one cocktail party every two weeks. Call me in sixty days.

This is not the sort of activity that we typically consider within the scope of medical care. We would not expect Blue Cross to pay for it or ask that medical insurance provide for such expenditures. Yet no dimension of life falls outside the realm of our physical, psychological, and social well-being; if the World Health Organization's definition of health set the scope of medical authority, the treatment described above would be uncontroversial.

It is time for a literary interlude. The passage is from *Oblomov*, a splendid novel by the nineteenth-century Russian Goncharov, who, lamentably, seems best noted for not being Dostoevsky. In this scene we see Oblomov facing the question of whether to get out of bed—a major decision which he ponders for nearly a hundred pages. He is visited by his physician, whose remarks illuminate our concern with the scope of the physician's legitimate authority. The physician speaks first:

"If you go on living in this climate for another two or three years, lying around, and eating rich, heavy food . . . you're going to die of a stroke."
Oblomov was startled. "What am I to do? Tell me, for God's sake."
"Do what other people do—go abroad."

Oblomov here pleads that his financial circumstances won't allow that at present, and the physician replies:

"Never mind, never mind, that's no affair of mine; my duty is to tell you that you must change your way of life, the place, the air, occupation, everything— everything. . . . Go to Kissingen, or to Ems," the doctor said. "Spend June and July there, drink the waters; then go to Switzerland or the Tyrol, take the grape cure. . . ."
"The Tyrol! How awful! . . . But what about my plan for the reorganization of my estate? Good heavens, Doctor, I'm not a block of wood, you know."
"Well, it's up to you. My business is simply to warn you. You must be on your guard against passions, too. They hinder the cure. You should try to amuse yourself by riding, dancing, moderate exercise in the fresh air, pleasant conversation, especially with ladies, so that your heart is only moderately stimulated and by pleasant sensations." . . .
"Anything more?"
"As for reading or writing—God forbid! Rent a villa facing south, with plenty of flowers; have lots of music and ladies around you . . ."
"What sort of food?"
"Avoid meats, all fish or fowl, also starchy foods and fat. You may have light bouillon, vegetables, but be on your guard: there is cholera almost everywhere now, so you must be very cautious. You may walk eight hours a day. . . ."
"Good Lord," Oblomov groaned.
"Finally," the doctor concluded, "spend the winter in Paris, and amuse yourself in the whirl of life. Don't think: go from the theatre to a ball, a masquerade, go out of town, surround yourself with friends, life, laughter—"
"Anything else?" Oblomov inquired with barely concealed annoyance.
"You might perhaps benefit from sea air. You can take a steamer to England, and from there to America. . . . If you carry this out exactly . . ."

"Certainly, certainly, without fail," replied Oblomov sarcastically. . . . The doctor went out, leaving Oblomov in a pitiful state. He closed his eyes, put both hands to his head, curled up in a ball in his chair, and sat there neither seeing nor feeling anything.[4]

What has the doctor told Oblomov to do? To become someone else! He has taken the WHO definition of health seriously. If that definition were correct, and if physicians can give orders with respect to health, then physicians could give orders with respect to every dimension of life. It becomes important, therefore, to clarify the physician's proper business and to understand what does and what does not fall within the scope of legitimate medical authority. So the sense in which medical practice is a puzzling profession has deepened, with the puzzles about why physicians behave as they do replaced by the more fundamental puzzle about how they ought to behave.

We have already noted the conventional wisdom about what physicians ought to do. They ought to treat illness, to prolong life, to alleviate suffering to the extent they can. But such judgments are superficial and do not clarify how physicians ought to act in cases of moral dilemma. Indeed, these judgments can even lead physicians astray. To see that this is so, we will have to question these principles, asking what is valuable about life, what is bad about illness, what is wrong with dying. But that is work for later chapters. First, I want to consider a number of actual cases that show how things can go morally wrong in situations that on the surface may not seem to involve moral considerations at all.

Some years ago I was invited to speak in southern California; I proposed "Moral Mayhem in Modern Medicine" as the title of my public address— the title that heads this chapter. I later received a telephone call from someone at my host university who reported, with some embarrassment, that the title simply would not do in Orange County. I was asked to revise it, out of consideration for the university's delicate relations with the larger political community. No stranger to such agonies, I changed the title to "Moral Muddles in Modern Medicine." My remarks were the same, of course, but the university escaped having an inflammatory title advertised throughout the community.

Mayhem is a strong word. It refers to a species of assault, a criminal act. It is understandable that I was taken as threatening to deliver an antimedical diatribe. And to some extent what I have to say *is* critical of medical practice. Yet in the end my position is not hostile to the medical profession in general. There are many superb physicians who are exemplars both of technical skill and of moral integrity. My objective is to clarify the ingredients of such exemplary practice and to explore ways in which physicians, patients, and others together can make it more characteristic of the profession.

The notion of moral mayhem is metaphorical; mayhem literally is a physical act against the body of a person. By *moral mayhem* I mean a violation of the integrity of a person—an action that abuses a person in a way that will not bear scrutiny, that has no adequate justification, that is morally indefensible. Medical practice abounds with such actions.

I do not here refer to the horror stories that we all are familiar with from the news media. The *Times* (of London), for example, carried a story in the Spring of 1980 about a girl who was hospitalized for the removal of a cancerous eye, only to have the surgeons erroneously remove her good eye instead. Such criminally negligent incompetence is properly dealt with through the courts, and I will have little to say about it. It is subtler, more pervasive problems that I am after. The cases I will cite will therefore not be the sort of highly dramatic cases that make the pages of the newspaper. Instead, they will be far more routine episodes in clinical practice. Perhaps I should have called this chapter "Moral Mayhem in Mundane Medicine."

Consider this first case. An octogenarian approaching death with end-stage cancer was very uncomfortable despite having been given analgesic medication. Her son (and guardian) asked the physician if there was not some way to increase her comfort. The physician said. "I'm sorry, we're doing everything that can be done. But she can't last much longer; it's a matter of days at this point."

The son, a philosopher, went away pondering what he had been told but made it only across the street before turning back to see the physician again. "I'm sorry," he said. "That just isn't good enough. I want you to explain why."

The physician was thoughtful, sensitive, and patient. He replied, "Don't apologize. I want you to feel free to ask me questions at any time, here at the office or at home. Ask new questions as they occur to you, or ask the same question over again because sometimes people need to do that, too. Here's my home number; don't feel shy about calling me there if you think it will help." And then the physician gave a little lesson in clinical pharmacology.

"How much medication we can give is determined in part by the fact that any drug is also a poison. If it is a drug at all, it is toxic, and there is a delicate trade-off. What relieves the pain also suppresses the respiration and invites infection. We have to consider total body weight and basic strength. The primary risks are that we can suppress respiration to a point that will kill the patient or will invite an infection that will kill the patient. There are also problems of increasing dependency, of the patient needing the drug at shorter and shorter intervals and becoming increasingly addicted.''

The son thanked the physician and went as far as the elevator before turning back. He said, ''I think I understand what is going on now. I want you to understand that I'm the last person to advocate that what this society needs is terminally ill octogenarian pushers out on the streets. I recognize that as a general convention of clinical practice it makes sense to be cautious in the use of drugs. But in this case I don't see the sense; I don't see possible addiction as having any bearing. And as for suppressing respiration, where is it written that the malignancy has some sort of entitlement to be the cause of death, as if somehow the physician has an obligation to keep the patient alive until the malignancy has had time to cash in its claim? Why is it bad if she dies of a drug-induced respiratory failure if she's more comfortable in the meantime?'' The physician had no ready answer, and the son continued. ''I see two conflicting values here, the prolongation of life and the relief of suffering. I see a convention in medical practice of how to respond to such a conflict, a convention that dictates that the prolongation of life is a more fundamental and important value than the relief of suffering. I see a physician who knows how things are usually done and why they are usually done that way and who recognizes that it is best that they usually be done that way. And I see those conventions and principles of practice being applied here where they just don't fit. Prolongation of life is in general more important than relief of suffering, but in this case those two values in conflict should not be weighted in the usual way. In this case relief of suffering is a more important value than the prolongation of life. Not only have you assumed which value is the more important in this case and then imposed that value on your patient, but you've done it without being aware that you were doing it at all.''

The physician replied, ''You're right.'' And he changed the prescription. The patient became more comfortable but did not live much longer. I do not know what she died of or whether she was addicted to anything at the time. No one thought these were interesting questions.

This is not a case that involves a vital decision in any significant sense; it is a rather ordinary piece of medical business. Yet it is a case of the first importance because ethical decisions—that is, decisions about matters of basic value—were being made by the physician, albeit unwittingly, and imposed on the patient. Making such a decision was, in a sense, none of the physician's proper business. What the physician did in this case was to overstep the bounds of his competence, of his expertise, of his legitimate authority, not out of maliciousness, not out of an imperialistic attitude, not out of any desire to play God—anyone who has been close to medical practice must realize that in such circumstances the last thing that physicians are doing is playing anything—but because of a lack of moral sensitivity. The result was a kind of moral mayhem—an assault on the patient's right to be treated in accordance with the values she held (represented here through the agency of her son, who functioned as guardian), rather than values imposed on her from without. And this with a highly skilled physician, earnestly striving to serve his patients in the best possible way.

A second case came to my attention when I visited a hospital in San Francisco in 1979, but it could have been anywhere. A man who had been hospitalized as terminally ill was close to death; his blood pressure was practically nothing, and his brain wave was essentially flat. A resident physician asked a nurse to bring the materials for a Swan-Ganz line—a delicate diagnostic procedure involving threading a catheter into the heart. The nurse conferred with another nurse, and they agreed not to comply because there was no possible benefit to the patient. At their peril, they refused. But the chief resident and a more junior resident got the materials themselves and initiated the procedure about forty minutes before the patient died. During this time the patient's family was in the hospital but did not have access to the patient. I do not know whether they wanted to be with him for the last moments; in any case they did not have access to his room while the procedure was being done. The nurses were acutely distressed by this instance of physicians' performing an invasive procedure on a patient it could not help, solely in order to practice. Their distress increased when they discovered that the patient's account was charged $200 for the Swan-Ganz line. If the procedure is done, someone has to pay.

It took some courage and some threats; finally, the nurses' tenacious complaining caused the residents to be criticized and the charge to be removed from the patient's account. Those physicians had wanted to learn how to do a Swan-Ganz line, in the interest of better service to their future patients who could benefit from the procedure. They believed that their need to learn justified what they did. But they had not been taught anything appropriate to the making of a decision about what kinds of practicing are justifiable and what kinds are not. They had the power to make that decision in this situation, but they had no education or wisdom that enabled them to see that what they did was unwarranted assault on the patient's body. Further, it is important to recognize that the victims of inappropriate medical care are not always patients. As in this case, they can also be the patient's family; they can be ancillary staff—people working for and with physicians—they can be insurers; they can be those who are connected in any way with the episode. Although the patient was, in a sense, beyond the possibility of injury and suffered no physical or psychological distress as a result of the incident, the family's right of access was disregarded, the body of the patient was treated merely as learning material, and the patient's estate or insurers were almost burdened with a charge to pay for it all. Moreover, the nurses, who exhibited better sense and sensitivity than the physicians to whom they were subordinate, were pressured to be complicit in an undertaking they found repugnant. Although they resisted that pressure, and in the end did so without penalty, there was substantial psychic cost imposed on them along the way. Yet there is no evidence that the physicians intended or were aware of any of these factors.

There has been a tendency in recent writing about medicine toward glorification of the patient. No longer, we read, can the physician act as the sole authority on what is best for the patient; Oblomov's physician is a thing of the past, patients' rights are the standard of the day, and the patient and physician must be viewed henceforth as partners in a common venture, serving the medical interests of the patient. Indeed, on some accounts, the patient must be recognized as retaining all decision-making authority, with the physician serving in the role of adviser and provider of services only at the request and direction of the patient who has pondered the advice. These views, although excessive, are an understandable reaction to defects in the way medicine has been practiced. I am somewhat sympathetic to them. Yet they fail to take adequate account of an important point.

Physicians, on the whole, are brighter than average; medical schools tend to admit only those with high academic achievement, which is correlated with above-average intelligence. Among physicians, however, are the dishonest, greedy, insensitive, alcoholic, drug-addicted, generally incompetent, lazy, ill-trained, mentally unstable, deeply ignorant, and, once in a while, just plain stupid. This should be no surprise; the same is true of other professional groups, such as lawyers, political leaders, and the professoriate. Any large group, no matter how carefully selected at the outset, will include some who have one or more of these liabilities. Even if the initial screening allows into the profession no one with such deficiencies, the passage of time will introduce some of these problems into any community that starts without them.

The population of patients is considerably broader than that of physicians, and the range of characteristics that patients have is therefore even more diverse than the range of characteristics that physicians exhibit. Some patients are aggressive, uncooperative, and nasty. Some are depressed to the point of substantial dysfunction. Some are crippled by fear; others, by irrational optimism. Some are unimaginably ignorant, and some are hopelessly dim. These factors place constraints, sometimes of a severe sort, on the amount of responsibility that can be borne by patients and on what role it is reasonable to expect them to play in regard to their own treatment. We shall return to this issue later. But bear in mind the diversity of patient characteristics as you consider the next case.

An unmarried and uneducated woman gave birth to an acutely ill baby. Its survival was in doubt from the outset. On the third day after delivery the physician came in to see the mother. "I'm terribly sorry," he said. "Your baby didn't make it. We did everything we could, but it just wasn't enough. I'd like to do an autopsy, and I'll need your permission for that." The mother granted permission, later confirmed by her signing an appropriate form. The next morning the physician stopped in to see how she was doing and to discuss her release from the hospital.

"Oh, Doctor, I'm so glad to see you," she said. "I've been so upset and worried. They gave me pills, but I couldn't sleep much anyway. Tell me, how is my baby? Did the autopsy help?" The stunned physician realized at once how completely he had failed. He had then to explain to the woman that her baby was dead and to inform her that an autopsy is a postmortem examination often conducted to confirm a cause of death. Troubled by the episode, he related it to his resident, from whom I later heard the tale.

The mother's failure to understand the physician's message was due in part to the fact that she did not know what an autopsy is—but only in part. It was also due to the fact that she was not told that her baby had died. Rather, she was told only that the baby "didn't make it." Such euphemistic expressions are common in hospitals, where patients expire, pass away, terminate, transcend, cross over, give up the ghost, and fail to make it, but rarely, if ever, just plain die. Such language is defended as being, or intended to be, protective of the patients and their families, sparing them the harshness of more direct accounts of death. But the use of euphemistic language to refer to the deaths of patients is also self-protective on the part of the physicians and other health care providers,

to whom death represents defeat and who, like anyone else, find it distasteful to be the bearers of tragic tidings.

Even the physician's lack of explicitness would have gone unnoticed,
however, if the mother had understood that the request for permission to
do an autopsy could arise only because the baby had died. Instead, she
took the message to be that the usual treatments were unable to cure the
baby, so now it was necessary to try some special treatment that required
special permission. It wasn't clear what that treatment was, but it was
called an autopsy.

The physician assumed—perhaps reasonably but erroneously—that an
understanding of what an autopsy is was included in the background
information brought to bear by the mother on the situation. He would
surely have explained a portacaval shunt and would not likely have seen
any need to explain taking the baby's temperature. Between these extremes lie a host of procedures that may or may not be understood,
depending on the patient. The physician failed to communicate effectively with his patient because he did not know who she was. Had he taken
the time to find out, the problem would have been avoided, but only at
the cost of the time he had taken. It is easy, in this case, to fault the
physician for failure of communication, but that is because it is equally
easy to see how the problem could have been avoided. If the physician
had taken his role as an educator of the patient more seriously and had
filled it more responsibly, understanding would have been achieved. But
other cases are not so simple. Had the mother been suffering from severely
diminished capacity, rather than from easily correctable ignorance, it
might have been a much larger undertaking to get her to understand the
circumstances. In other kinds of cases, moreover, the information is far
more complex, and imparting it to some patients can be not merely
difficult but impossible. It is not easy to determine the extent to which
the physician has an obligation to function as educator of the patient in
circumstances in which doing so is unusually difficult or time-consuming,
nor is it entirely clear what constraints on treatment should follow from
the fact that the patient's understanding is flawed. These issues will
concern us in the chapter on informed consent.

The consent given by the mother to perform the autopsy was only a
procedural exercise. It was based on misunderstanding, and as a result,
the autopsy was done without the mother's having agreed to have such
an action performed. If we assume the validity of the consent requirement
in this circumstance, the mother's rights in regard to the body of her
dead child were clearly violated—even if she would readily have con-
sented on the basis of a correct understanding.

These cases, and others like them, illustrate the way in which day-to-day medical practice is laden with moral dimensions that are often unrecognized by both those providing and those receiving the medical care. When there is a question of whether to terminate a life, to transfuse a patient over that patient's objections, or to perform a lifesaving operation on a severely retarded child over the objections of the parents, there is no likelihood that moral dilemma will be missed. The circumstances in medical practice that cry out for moral clarification are legion and have become especially well known during the last decade. In such cases the effort to determine the right thing to do arises in response to a recognition that it is not clear which course of action is the right one. We will consider a number of situations of this kind later. The cases we have just considered are not like that, however. They are cases, instead, in which no moral dilemma is readily apparent. Yet they do challenge one's moral sensitivity, for they all are cases in which some violation of rights has occurred where no question of rights was recognized by the physicians as even arising. It is cases like these that constitute the fabric of medical practice, and it is therefore cases like these that I want to emphasize before going on to issues of more obvious moral interest.

Finally, this last example, which also came to my attention during a visit to a hospital. One issue in great dispute was the question of how to make decisions about long-term intensive care of newborns weighing less than 600 grams. There were cases which the nursing staff believed should be abandoned as hopeless, while the medical staff believed that maximum effort should be made to the last second. Such efforts incur tremendous costs—psychic costs to the nursing staff and the parents, possibly to the child itself, and economic costs. Although nothing in medical training equips physicians to make a well-informed judgment about which cases are appropriate for valiant intervention, the power structure in the hospital is such that physicians typically make the decision. This is a clear example in which the authority of the physician exceeds the scope of his expertise. But it would be a mistake to blame physicians too quickly for making decisions that they are in a position to make and that, after all, must be made. Rather, I want to raise a concern about the motivation with which such decisions are made.

The skills brought to bear in any intensive care unit are hard earned and demanding to exercise. There is an aesthetic appeal to the use of such skills. Two people, both of whom know both checkers and chess, are likely to play chess, not checkers. Skills that have been acquired at substantial personal cost are skills that people like to use; people who can do sophisticated things like to do them. There is an intrinsic payoff in satisfaction. State-of-the-art medical practice is highly sophisticated, and understandably, the people who can do it often find it a very beautiful thing to be doing. We should bear this in mind as we consider the motivation behind some of the decisions that are made in medical practice. There is a common view that medical decisions are motivated solely by a consideration of the interests of the patient, but it is naïve to accept the claim at face value. The motivation behind medical decisions is complex, and it is not even obvious that the interests of the patient should be, or can be, the only operative consideration. Still, it is worth worrying, given the spectacular power of the position in which the physician is placed, whether the motivation of medical decisions is adequately understood. For when a decision is made for reasons that are not solely a function of patient interests, there is a risk that the interests of the patient are being subordinated to some other value, and the result may be violation of the patient's legitimate claims.

It is well known that in morally troubling cases physicians have enormous power to affect the lives and welfare of other people. We have seen that even in situations that do not appear initially to be morally puzzling, physicians play a role that can easily involve them in a violation of the legitimate claims of their patients and others. We have moved from a consideration of what physicians do to a puzzlement about what they ought to be expected to do, and we have seen that what they do can be morally charged even in apparently straightforward circumstances. It is time to consider in more detail some of the morally troubling aspects of the interactions between physicians and patients.

2

Medical Mistakes

I HAVE REFERRED TO THE RISK involved in being a patient—to the fact that physicians make many mistakes. I want now to take a closer look at how medical errors come about and to consider how doctors, patients, and the public can deal with them more reasonably. Errors in medical practice are intensely feared by physicians and patients alike. Patients who suffer damage at the hands of their physicians often seek compensation through malpractice suits, and physicians and hospitals view such suits as perhaps the only outcomes to be more earnestly avoided than even the errors from which they presumably arise. Defensive medicine, in which physicians make treatment decisions not strictly on the basis of what is best for the patient but also in part on the basis of what will establish the most defensible record of physician behavior, is on the increase. Patients thus must sometimes bear the discomfort, inconvenience, cost, and risk of tests the physician does not see as medically necessary but has ordered so that the record will demonstrate impeccable treatment should the need later arise. Malpractice insurance rates soar, physicians strike in reaction, legislatures intervene, and in the end the quality of health care suffers from the absence of a clear understanding of what medical error is, how it arises, to what extent it is avoidable, when it is culpable, and what relationship it should bear to compensation for harm. It is this cluster of issues I wish to consider.

A few facts seem clear at the outset. Medical error not only occurs but seems to some extent unavoidable. Some of it seems innocent even when serious damage results, but other errors seem clearly culpable. The harm that results from medical error seems sometimes, but not always, to warrant compensation, and errors in practice, whether or not they cause harm, seem sometimes, but not always, to warrant sanctions. It would be useful to be able to distinguish between culpable and innocent error and to lessen the obscurity surrounding the relationships among harm, culpability, compensation, and sanctions.

Too often we approach these matters with concepts and categories that have developed in other areas, without reflecting carefully enough on whether they best suit the issues in clinical practice. For example, lawyers apparently assume that legislators and the courts are competent to determine when medical error is culpable and, correspondingly, when patients are entitled to compensation, by applying the general principles with which our legal system handles torts. The reaction of the medical profession has normally been to claim prerogatives of professional jurisdiction in response, arguing that it is in the best interests of quality health care for physicians themselves to monitor the behavior of their colleagues, make judgments, and impose sanctions through processes internal to the profession. The public response is often to accuse the medical profession of a conspiracy of silence, aimed at preventing anyone outside the profession from learning what actually happened when there is a suspicion of medical blundering—justifying the conspiracy with the pretense that only physicians have the necessary knowledge to understand and assess the behavior of physicians and to determine and apply corrective or punitive sanctions where there has been a violation of the standards of performance within the profession.

Recently, however, the courts have challenged the traditional standards for evaluating medical practice. Whereas the standard of acceptability had been based on what was customary practice within the local medical community, that standard has come under pressure of a variety of sorts. Some decisions have favored judging a physician's performance against the standard of what specialists of the relevant sort do on a national basis, allowing for both the standard approaches to treatment and the possibility of a respected and responsible minority view about treatment. And the recent *Canterbury* decision has moved the standard even farther away from the traditional, medically dominated one. According to *Canterbury*, the information provided to a patient must be not merely whatever a responsible physician would typically provide but what a reasonable patient would want.[1] So the physicians' efforts to police their own activities according to their own internal standards are meeting increasingly effective resistance.

Medicine is an art based on, although transcending, the findings of medical science. It will be useful, therefore, to step back from clinical practice a bit, to consider the place of error in purely scientific endeavors. At any moment a scientist's standards are necessarily set by the present state of the discipline, and there will be limits in the extent to which even the greatest thinker can make progress—limits resulting from partial ignorance about the subject matter of the discipline. Indeed, if *everything* were known about a given area of science, all *scientific* activity in that area would cease. How could you possibly do research in an area you completely understood? Of course, work might continue on the practical *applications* of that knowledge. Where there is scientific activity, there must be partial ignorance—the ignorance that is a precondition for scientific progress. And since ignorance is a precondition of progress, where there is a possibility of progress, there is also a possibility of error. This ignorance of what is not yet known is the permanent state of all science and is a source of error even when there is flawless adherence to the norms of methodology, care, and honesty that characterize impeccable scientific inquiry. Of course, those norms can be violated; a scientist can willfully misrepresent results in an effort to beat competitors into print or can negligently make errors in calculation that result in an erroneous conclusion.

In one traditional view, all errors in science arise either from the limitation of the present state of the discipline—that is, from ignorance— or from willfulness or negligence of the scientist—that is, from ineptitude of one sort or another. This view of ignorance and ineptitude as the only sources of error has been transmitted from the pure to the applied sciences and hence, more specifically, from medical science to medical practice— the clinical application of what is learned by medical science. For example, if the physician prescribes a drug that unexpectedly has disastrous side effects for the patient, then either the limits of pharmaceutical and physiological knowledge are to blame or the physician was negligent—that is, failed to obtain and act in accordance with the best knowledge available. On the very reasonable assumption that the physician did not bring about the side effects willfully, one or the other of these two causes must have been operative. Where a surgeon is involved, lack of technical skill may also be a factor. But such lacks themselves arise from the same two sources of error: Either they spring from the general level of the art— the surgical technique in question has just not advanced far enough, in which case lack of surgical skill compares to scientific ignorance—or the particular surgeon has been negligent either in acquiring or in exercising the requisite available skills. But this view of the origins of error fails to take adequate account of the fact that clinical medicine is an art directed to the good of individuals. To understand the significance of this fact, we have to consider briefly the question of what science is about.

For natural science, the objects of knowledge are typically taken to be the properties or characteristics of objects classified by kinds and the generalizations that link those properties. The scientist looks for lawlike relationships between properties, such as molecular structure and conductivity. Individual objects are of interest only as the bearers of general properties; scientists want to know how interferon proteins *in general* behave, not just how this *particular* bit of interferon protein behaves, or how amino acids of a particular sort are formed, not just how a particular sample of the acid was formed. But something important escapes notice in this view of science.

Much of the time we are interested in individual objects—some of them complex composites of other individuals—rather than in general principles or laws about a whole class of objects. I have in mind such individuals as a particular planet, salt marsh, horse, hurricane, or person. Every individual object has the characteristics that it has only because of the operation of physical and chemical mechanisms, and sometimes our interest in an object can be satisfied on the basis of our understanding of the physics and chemistry that are involved. Some objects—ice cubes and molecules are notable examples—are such that nearly everything we want to know about them can be explained in terms of the relevant mechanisms discovered by the natural and biological sciences. And the laws that describe their behavior are laws we can accept as perfectly reliable. Thus, roasted ice cubes always melt, and we can predict with complete assurance that any particular ice cube we roast will behave like any other—it will melt. There is little diversity of any sort that interests us where ice cubes are concerned. Each one, roughly speaking, is just like any other. Of course, if we are competing for the world bartending championship, our perspective changes, and we may then be very interested in the shape and mineral content of individual ice cubes.

So sometimes we are interested in an object not as an *example* of the objects of that kind, but as a *particular individual* that is distinctive. For instance, sometimes we want to know not just how hurricanes in general behave but what a particular hurricane will do next. Hurricanes interact continuously with a variety of uncontrollable environmental factors. No hurricane is quite like any other. Everything that happens in and to a hurricane, of course, is governed by scientific laws. But we never know in advance what historically specific interactions will influence the hurricane we are interested in—for example, because of melting icebergs, changes in the temperature of deep-sea waters, and so on. So we are never completely sure what scientific laws will be relevant in what ways to the behavior of the hurricane we are concerned about.

In order to have such knowledge, we would need to know all the relevant scientific laws, and we would also need to know in detail what the behavior would be of each potential influence on the particular hurricane. We would have to have a perfect understanding of the polar ice cap and of the Gulf Stream. But these, too, are particular objects interacting with their larger environments, which include among other things the very hurricane we seek to understand. Indeed, we cannot have perfect knowledge of our hurricane without a complete understanding of all the laws that describe natural processes and also a complete description of the state of the world. In short, perfect knowledge of that one particular hurricane is impossible short of omniscience. If we make an error in predicting what the hurricane will do, it may result from ignorance of the relevant scientific laws, or it may be due to the vagaries of the environmental context in which the hurricane operates—a context that is radically different from the contexts of laboratory science in its complexity and in the impossibility of isolating it from outside factors. No degree of meteorological knowledge will enable us in actual practice to do more than score a certain degree, though perhaps an increasingly high degree, of predictive success with hurricanes.

Now consider smallpox vaccination. Before such vaccination was discontinued, 1 person in 1,200 would experience a dangerous and perhaps fatal reaction to the vaccination. Although there must be reasons why some people succumb—factors that distinguish them from the majority, who are unharmed by the vaccination—no one knows what those factors are. So we cannot accept the generalization that vaccinated people, even of a certain sort, will be unharmed by the vaccination. We do have confidence in the claim that *for the most part*, vaccinated people suffer no ill effects, despite the few instances of illness or even death. What, then, can we predict of an individual about to be vaccinated? Of course, the effect of the vaccine on him will be determined by the laws of science, his condition, and perhaps the way in which he interacts with his environment subsequent to the vaccination. But we do not know *all* the relevant laws and conditions; our knowledge of this individual is limited, and our predictive ability is therefore constrained. We can have reasonable, scientifically based expectations held with a high degree of confidence, but no more is available to us than that. Yet more would be needed to eliminate *entirely* the possibility of causing harm by using the vaccine.

What is typically important to the scientist—including the medical scientist—is general knowledge, not the distinctive features of a particular molecule, crystal, or other entity. The scientist does have an interest in such entities, but it is an interest in what they have in common with others of the same kind that typifies research. Thus, principles of crystal formation or solubility are inferred from the observable characteristics of diverse particular crystals, but the differences among such crystals are not to the point; it is their similarities that support scientific generalizations. In contrast, what is important to the meteorologist, navigator, or veterinary surgeon is primarily an understanding of particular, individual hurricanes, cloud formations, or cows, and thus, what is distinctive about them as individuals is of crucial importance. How such individuals differ from one another in their diversity thus becomes as important as the characteristics they commonly share with others of their kind.

Experience of a single entity over time is typically necessary for an understanding of that entity as an individual in all its distinctiveness; its distinctive *individual* characteristics will not be inferable simply from what is known about the general, commonly shared properties of objects of the same kind. Indeed, it might take more than superficial observation over time to increase significantly one's understanding of the distinctive properties of a particular object. It might take a careful examination of that object—possibly an examination of an intrusive or even destructive sort. If we knew what to look for to identify the 1 person in 1,200 who would fall victim to smallpox vaccination, the test to identify those persons at risk might be far more deadly than the vaccination itself!

Because we often cannot achieve perfect understanding of particular, individual objects even on the basis of scientific research and examination of the particular object, the best possible judgment about an object of our interest may turn out to be erroneous—not merely because science has not progressed far enough, or because the scientist has been willful or negligent, but because of the necessary limitations of our knowledge of those particular objects in which we are interested. What underscores that necessity is the fact that in the case of exceedingly complex objects like people, which interact with their environments in complex ways, our ability to improve our predictive power about them is limited by their fragility—by the fact that in the process of learning more about them as individuals, we can damage or destroy them before we have learned as much about them as it would take to make our practical judgments about them more secure.

Recognition of this element of necessary fallibility disposes of that twofold classification of the sources of error discussed above. Error may indeed arise from the present state of scientific ignorance or from willfulness or negligence. But it may also arise precisely from this third factor, the necessary fallibility of our knowledge of particular fragile and complex individuals. Two consequences follow concerning the practice of medicine.

The first concerns the research of medicine. It is not common clinical practice outside academic medical centers and teaching hospitals to keep full and systematic records of medical or surgical error. (For a particularly illuminating study of how errors are handled in the training of surgeons, see Charles Bosk's fascinating treatise *Forgive and Remember*.[2]) Physicians often flinch from even identifying error in clinical practice, let alone recording it, perhaps because they are themselves inclined to hold the view that error arises from either ignorance or ineptitude. But without detailed records of erroneous diagnoses and prognoses, of unpredicted side effects, of failure of treatment, and the like, we cannot build the empirical basis necessary for any adequate theory of the limitations of the predictive power of clinical medicine, nor are we likely to learn as much as we otherwise could about how to avoid the errors that are eliminable. (Physicians are not alone in their lack of systematic attention to their errors; political scientists and economists, for example, also seem not to maintain systematic records of their own false predictions and rarely refer to them in public utterance.)

The second consequence is the one I want to emphasize. It concerns the physician's liability for error and the patient's attitude toward the physician. At present the typical patient is encouraged to believe that his or her physician will not make a mistake, even though what the physician does may not achieve the desired medical objectives and even though it cannot be denied that every physician does make some mistakes. This belief is reinforced by the absence of an adequate public understanding of medical error. Yet it is a false confidence. The high incidence of iatrogenic illness constitutes a medical and health policy problem of enormous proportions, well recognized within government agencies and much of the medical profession, but only dimly suspected by the public. Despite the fact that clinical medicine does more good than harm, there is still a substantial probability that a patient will suffer from medical error.

It is just here that the moral dimensions of medicine as an applied science concerned with particular individuals become important. Patients and the public have to learn to recognize, accept, and respond reasonably to the necessary fallibility of the individual physician. The physician-patient relationship is one in which mistakes necessarily will be made, sometimes culpably, sometimes because of the state of development of medical science, but sometimes, ineliminably, because of the inherent limitations in the predictive powers of an enterprise concerned essentially with the flourishing of particular, complex, fragile individuals. The patient and the public must understand that medical science is committed to the patient's flourishing and that the treatment of the patient is itself a *part* of that science and not a mere application of it. The patient thus must understand that clinical intervention aims at his good but may do him harm. Indeed, the familiar distinction between therapeutic medicine and medical research seems utterly to break down. Since the effect of any therapeutic intervention on a particular patient is always to some extent uncertain, no matter how much is known about the general characteristics of interventions of that type, every therapeutic intervention is an experiment in regard to the well-being of that individual patient.

All experiments involve the possibility of failure, in the sense that the expected or hypothesized outcome may not occur, whereas other outcomes, unintended and not usually specifiable in advance, may occur. Thus, the possibility of failure, and even of damaging failure, is linked unavoidably to the notion of experimentation and, therefore, to the practice of clinical medicine.

It should seem obvious at this point that it is wrong to link the notion of injury directly to the notion of culpability. A physician may damage a patient without violating the canons of impeccable practice. A common response to such outcomes is humility in regard to the state of medical knowledge, but what is more appropriate is humility in regard to the richness and diversity of individuals, regardless of the state of medical science. Even the hypothetical clinical practitioner who is fully informed of all the general principles that apply to medical practice—not merely present medical knowledge but even to the extent that represents the aspirations of medical research—would be far from infallible. He would stand humbled by the mysteries of individual diversity and would know that an inquiry into the distinctiveness of each individual patient is an essential ingredient of good practice. Inquire as he might, there would always remain the prospect of his harming the patient whose well-being is in his trust, for even that inquiry itself, that effort to understand the distinctiveness of the patient, could be damaging. And if such is the plight of our hypothetical physician, actual physicians are also limited by an irredeemably inadequate understanding of the individuals in their care.

Good clinical practice has always required respect for individual distinctiveness; hence the importance of the individual medical history as a part of competent practice. But the point here is not simply that regard for the particular individual is essential to good medical practice; rather, it is that knowledge about the individual patient is always and necessarily potentially inadequate in the sense that damaging error may result even from conscientious, well-motivated clinical intervention by even the best-informed physicians.

It follows that injury is no proof of culpability. Physicians should recognize this point and become far less reluctant to acknowledge, systematize, and learn from injury. But that also requires a widened willingness on the part of patients to lower their expectations about what physicians can reasonably be expected to accomplish and to refrain from assuming physician culpability even in the disappointment or despair that attends iatrogenic injury.

The first reaction of physicians invited to dispense with the mask of infallibility is often a humane alarm at the insecurity that a frank admission of medical fallibility might engender in the patient. But consider whether the present situation, in which the expectations of patients are so very often disappointed during medical treatment, is not a greater source of insecurity. It is certainly one key source of malpractice suits. Indeed, a rewriting of the laws on malpractice and compensation for iatrogenic injury should acknowledge the inevitability of medical error and make the process for assessing malpractice quite different from what it is now.

The question of what constitutes culpable malpractice, like the question of what constitutes injurious medical activity, is of fundamental importance in the determination of policy governing the relationships among culpability, sanctions, and compensation. Whether a medical action is an instance of malpractice should be seen as a question not of whether the action had undesirable consequences, but of whether the action was justifiable as performed—whether it followed the canons of good medical practice. That does not depend on the actual consequences of the intervention in question. The canons of good medical practice will depend heavily on what has worked in the past and on the degree to which a flexible range of physician judgment in clinical circumstances tends to be conducive to a good medical result. Once those canons are specified, however, whether or not they have been honored becomes a question of empirical fact, quite different from the question of the subsequent well-being of the patient.

I do not mean to suggest that it is a simple matter to specify the canons of good medical practice. On the contrary, the description of what should count as good medical practice is exceedingly difficult. I shall have more to say about what the criteria of good medical practice should include when I offer a characterization below of the good doctor. For now, suffice it to say that the canons of good practice should cover both the requirements of technical competence and the requirements of moral sensitivity.

A profession concerned with minimizing malpractice should then specify as well as possible the canons of good practice; it should require, as an inherent part of good practice, the maintenance of accurate medical records, including records of error and injury; and it should adopt some effective mechanisms to identify culpable error. (Greater use of computer-based information systems could play a significant role here, provided that the medical profession's misgivings about such systems can be overcome.) There should be procedures of due process and sanctions for the performance of culpable error. But no injury to a patient should be required as part of the proof of any malpractice claim. If a violation of good medical practice is of a kind that is likely to cause injury that proper treatment would avoid, or constitutes an assault on the patient's dignity, the absence of actual resulting injury is simply not material to the claim that malpractice has occurred.

In this respect, malpractice is properly viewed as a formal violation of rules, procedures, and canons of practice—what philosophers describe as a deontological offense, in contrast with an action's being considered an offense only if it actually leads to bad consequences. There is a broad spectrum of degrees of seriousness of such offenses and, correspondingly, of appropriate sanctions, ranging from the most gentle—privately calling the error to the attention of the offending physician—to the most extreme, at least within the profession—revocation of license to practice. In this conception, the primary burden for discovering malpractice, bringing charges, supporting claims, and imposing sanctions falls not to the individual injured patient, but to those who are concerned with the integrity of the medical profession, including perhaps most prominently the practitioners of medicine themselves.

Injury at the hands of physicians is quite another matter. Having seen that physician culpability is independent of actual injury to the patient—in the sense that there can be malpractice without injury and injury without malpractice—we need to reassess the relationship of injury to compensation. That is, we need to reconsider the formulation of a policy for societal response to iatrogenic injury.

I will not argue for any specific policy here. That would involve a discussion of social values and social decision making that would take us too far afield. I will simply note that any policy that is to be acceptable must abandon the idea of a direct conceptual linkage from physician-caused injury through physician liability to entitlement to compensation enforced through the mechanisms of law.

Indeed, one of the weakest features of current medical practice is the absence of effective patient grievance procedures that involve milder measures than reliance on the courts or the threat of litigation. The best physicians have relationships with their patients that encourage open communication, including the discussion of discontents the patient may have. But far too many physicians leave the unsatisfied patient no choices other than to suffer in silence, to seek medical care elsewhere, or to sue. Both physicians and patients would stand to benefit, I believe, by the introduction of more effective and systematic ways for the consumers of medical care to be assertive about their discontents, without thereby alienating their physicians to the point of making good therapeutic relationships impossible. A greater mutual acknowledgment of what sorts of errors arise in medical practice, how they come about, what their connection is with injury and with affront, and what can be done about them would surely make an important contribution to improved relationships between doctors and their patients.

If physicians were perfect, both in having perfect medical knowledge and in making perfect medical decisions on the basis of that knowledge, there would be little basis for patients to be discontent. But that is not the real world. Instead, the practice of medicine is exceedingly difficult in a variety of ways, and patients are often unhappy, for justifiable and unjustifiable reasons, with what their physicians do. The reality of risk and the possibility of error make it crucial for physicians to be conscientious in the way they explain proposed treatments to their patients and in the way they involve their patients in making decisions about what should be done. And even here there is the possibility of error, for it is not easy to decide how much a patient should be told, nor is it easy to decide on the extent to which a patient's autonomy should be respected in medically difficult situations. Our consideration of mistakes in medical practice thus leads us to problems surrounding the doctrine of informed consent and the value of patient autonomy.

3

Informed Consent and Patient Autonomy

THE CASE of the misunderstood autopsy, described in chapter 1, illustrates that a patient can appear to the physician to have given consent to a medical procedure when the patient actually does not understand at all what the procedure involves. A key ingredient in the way things can go wrong is ignorance on the part of the patient. But sometimes the patient is quite sophisticated. Consider this actual case. A woman was hospitalized a few years ago for a biopsy to determine the character of a small lump in her breast. She knew that vigorous controversy existed within the medical profession about the various ways of dealing with malignancy— ranging from radiation and chemotherapy without surgery to radical mastectomy—and she knew that some physicians, but not all, favored performing a mastectomy immediately upon a diagnosis of malignancy, while the patient was still under the anesthesia that was employed in order to do the biopsy. She hoped for a negative finding, feared a positive finding, and resolved that if malignancy were found, she would look carefully into the therapeutic options, in consultation with several physicians, before deciding which treatment to elect. Since she knew that treatment standards in such cases varied to some extent from city to city, she saw the matter as involving a certain amount of fashion, and she determined that in a matter of such importance to her, the decision would be made on the most rational grounds that she could establish, rather than on the basis of the city she happened to be in. Not everyone approved of her resolve, but no one doubted her right to take such a stand.

The woman had recently suffered a marital separation. At best, such an experience is emotionally disorienting; at worst, it can be shattering. She knew that the truth about any marriage is elusive and that the truth about a failed marriage is often most distorted to those whose marriage it is. Struggling to gain a clear perspective on her circumstances, she had gone to a psychiatrist. But he saw her as having a sound and balanced sense of herself and her circumstances, with no need for psychiatric treatment. Nonetheless, when she later was admitted to the hospital for the biopsy, she replied to an inquiry on an admissions form that she had seen a psychiatrist recently. Unbeknownst to her, she was then classified as a patient with a psychiatric history. In consequence, although she was unaware of it at the time, she was given a double-strength dose of soporific medication at bedtime the night before the biopsy. Patients with psychiatric histories have difficulty sleeping, in the judgment of that hospital, and its convention of practice was to give them, automatically, a more powerful sleeping pill than is given to other patients. An hour after the medication the woman was nearly asleep. A surgical resident appeared with a consent form for her to sign. She had trouble reading it but had the presence of mind and fortitude to send the resident away, telling him to leave the form and return in the morning, when she would be clear-headed. And in the morning, when she examined the consent form, she saw that her signing it would have authorized the hospital and medical staff to perform any procedure that in their judgment would be in her best interest. She rejected the form, negotiated a revision that gave more limited consent, and then underwent the biopsy procedure.

The ethical issue raised by this case is that of informed consent. A large and growing literature on the subject gives testimony to its importance and to the disputes surrounding it. I do not propose to resolve those disputes here; I do propose to explore them as a way of gaining further understanding of medical transactions. The questions I will consider directly are these: What is informed consent, why is it required, can the requirement be met, and is it an aid or impediment to good medical care? Each of these questions gives rise to controversy.

Much medical treatment is in some way assaultive, as we have seen. Some treatment that one would stop short of calling assaultive is nonetheless limiting of the patient's freedom of action. Such interventions on the part of the physicians in the lives of their patients require justification; it is important to seek clarity both about why justification is necessary and how it is possible. If individual persons had no rights or freedoms except as bestowed upon them by the state of which they were citizens, then the state could decide that individual citizens had no proper voice in the management of their own medical affairs, that the health of the citizenry is a concern of the state, and that individuals must submit unquestioningly to medical decisions made about them by physicians. That we reject such a position is at once a philosophical point about the dignity of persons as worthy of respect as individuals and a political point about the relationship between the individual and the body politic. We who believe in the principles of liberal democracy believe not that persons exist to serve the state, but rather that political structures have their justification ultimately in the benefits that accrue to individuals; in this matter we take a position not always dominant throughout political history. But it is a fundamental underpinning of the cultural traditions in the context of which American medical institutions have developed. And it has important consequences for the way medicine can justifiably be practiced.

If this were a treatise on the foundations of political philosophy, it would be appropriate here to defend, rather than merely to affirm, the principle that individual persons are each, separately, of moral significance, worthy of respect, the bearers of basic rights and freedoms, and hence the final arbiters—subject to very limited constraints—of their own fates. Such a defense is not easy, however, for the principle represents so basic a commitment about the nature of persons that it would be difficult to find a more fundamental principle in terms of which to defend it, without relying on claims which themselves stand in even greater need of defense. In this respect, a commitment to human dignity is like a commitment to rationality; one who does not share it stands almost beyond the realm of discourse. I will not defend the position here but will take it as given, noting for now only that each of the theories of morality we will consider in chapter 5—despite their diversity—rests on the view that individual interests and individual rights are the basic ingredients out of which the structure of morality is built.

Because we respect individuals, we subscribe to what has been called the Principle of Autonomy, the view that individuals are entitled to be and do as they see fit, so long as they do not violate the comparable rights of others. No person is to be merely the instrument of another person's plans; no person is to be treated in a manner that is blind to the plans, desires, and values that are the fabric of his or her life and identity. Roughly speaking, we believe that it is obligatory to leave people alone, unless we have powerful reasons for not doing so. Such reasons arise with remarkable frequency, however.

Because we care about the well-being of individual persons, we also grant a prominent place in the structure of our moral outlook to a second principle, often called the Principle of Beneficence. That principle, simply stated, holds that one ought to do good. Doing good means benefiting people, helping them, acting—out of respect for their interests—in a way that serves their interests. It is this principle that is typically invoked as the justification for overriding the Principle of Autonomy, when we limit someone else's freedom in order to achieve what we see as being his or her own good.

Parents, obviously, do this as a matter of course. For that reason the phenomenon has come to be known as paternalism (why not *parentalism* one might well ask), and the philosophical and medical literature is laced through with lively debates about what grounds adequately justify paternalistic intervention in the life of another. For the parent of a small child, there is no issue; the parent has a responsibility to act in the interest of the child. If a four-year-old rushes toward the street in pursuit of a ball without regard for the oncoming traffic, the responsible parent does not say, "There is an aspect of your behavior that is imprudent in my judgment; please allow me to try to persuade you to change your approach to the problem of the ball." The parent grabs the child, obliterating its autonomy, and snatches it to safety. The action is classically paternalistic, but no one would doubt its justifiability.

The situation is quite different, however, if the relationship is not between parent and child, but between two adults. Suppose that you have taken a lover whom I rightly believe to be bad for you and, further, that I have tried earnestly but with no success to convince you by rational argument that my point of view is correct. Am I then justified in active intervention in your relationship—hiding your car keys as you prepare for an assignation, writing each of you an offensive letter over the other's signature, and the like? We are strongly inclined to say that such actions are unjustifiable; that the mere fact that I am right about the relationship's being bad for you does not entitle me to intervene beyond trying to convince you that you ought, autonomously and for your own reasons, to end it yourself. Even if the issue involves a life-threatening situation— for instance, your decision to take up skydiving or smoking or to become a mercenary—I must in the end respect your right to choose for yourself.

If we hesitate in making this judgment, it is likely that we realize that special circumstances that alter the situation may prevail. Perhaps I am your guardian, your brother, or your spouse. If there is some special relationship between us, then my responsibilities and my rights in regard to you may take on a different cast, and what under other circumstances would be unwarranted may be justified after all. The physician, for example, has a special relationship to the patient; perhaps, as a consequence, it is appropriate or even obligatory for the physician to act in a paternalistic way toward the patient.

For parents, it is a challenge to overcome the responsibilities of having young children, through a period of transition that sees paternalistic action diminish in harmony with the increasing autonomy and responsibility of the child. Adolescence is particularly demanding for both child and parent largely because it is the time of greatest alteration of roles, as the child often outgrows the need for paternalistic intervention more effectively than the parent outgrows the habit of paternalistic intervention. In medical practice, too, setting the limits of paternalism is difficult, as the well-intentioned physician, like the chronic parent, can easily override the autonomy of the patient in the interest of doing good without due regard for the question of whether the instance of paternalistic intervention is justifiable. This is not to say that patient autonomy is, or should be, supreme. It is to say that there is a problem about identifying its proper limits, just as there is a problem about identifying the proper scope of the physician's legitimate authority. These two problems are obviously related, and they come together over the issue of informed consent.

The doctrine of informed consent is simple and clear on the surface. Physicians do the sorts of things to their patients that people in general cannot justifiably do to one another. If the patient understands what the physician proposes to do and, thus informed, consents to its being done, then the medical intervention is not imposed on the patient in violation of the patient's autonomy; rather, that medical intervention is properly viewed as a service provided to the patient at the patient's request. Not only does this procedure of gaining informed consent respect the patient's autonomy, but it also protects the physician against the charge of imposing treatment on a patient who did not want that treatment—it protects the physician, in other words, against the charge of assault. On the face of it, the requirement should be applauded on all sides. But it is not.

In order to see why, we need to gain a clearer idea of what informed consent actually is. Obviously, it has two parts; informing and consenting. The physician does the former; the patient, the latter. At either point things can go wrong.

A common error to which professors are prone is instructive to consider here: the assumption that teaching is accomplished if the information to be taught is presented in a clear and accurate way. Ofttimes we tend to be so taken with the accuracy, insight, and eloquence of our lectures that it takes reading student examinations to remind us how far short we have fallen of achieving the goal, which is, after all, not to perform an entertainment that gives the impression to us or to the students of being uplifting or edifying, but to bring about specific changes in the minds of the students. (If we do not succeed in changing the interiors of the students' heads, then our universities are simply overpriced day care facilities for late adolescents, no matter how much illusion of edification there may be.) But teaching something to a student means bringing it about that the student understands it, and that may require more than simply saying it, no matter how well. Informed consent can go wrong in the informing because informing, like any other sort of teaching, is often harder to accomplish than one expects.

An attending surgeon sought permission to repair the heart of a newborn baby. In explaining to the mother that there was a leakage from one side of the heart to the other, he drew this diagram:

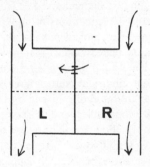

"The heart," he said, "has two chambers, the left and the right. In your baby's case, the two sides are connected by a little hole that lets blood get through from one side to the other. That's no good, and if we don't fix it, your baby won't do well at all and may not live. But that's the kind of problem we can fix. We just go in there and sew up that little hole, so the blood stays on the side it should be on. Then your baby will probably have a completely normal life."

Later the surgical resident went to see the mother to confirm her understanding of what was being done and why. He asked her if she understood; she said she did. "I want to make sure," he said, "so I'd like you to tell me in your own words what the problem is."

"The problem," she replied, "is that my baby's got a square heart."

In this case the attending physician's efforts to explain had been conscientious, and some might argue that an adequate level of understanding had been achieved. It is enough, they could hold, that the woman understood there was some problem with the heart which the physician saw as serious but operable and that on such an understanding, she gave consent. But whether or not an adequate level of consent was achieved in this case, the resident was surprised by the distortion of information that was reflected in the mother's account of the problem, and he learned from the encounter how differently a patient and a physician can interpret the same language and visual images. Human physiology is largely a mystery to most people even at the level of gross anatomy. The woman in this case reacted more strongly to the drawing—which conflicted with her conception of what heart-shaped objects look like—than she did to the physician's words because of her misconception of human anatomy and her unexpectedly literal interpretation of the drawing. If the original physician had asked the mother to explain the problem in her own words, as the resident later did, he might have learned at the outset how limited a level of understanding he had achieved.

It is not just unusual interpretations or unexpected ignorance that can impede understanding. Heightened anxiety associated with illness, the effects of medication, the regression that is commonly exhibited by patients, the mechanisms of denial, and many other factors can also interfere, and commonly do. Recent empirical studies have shown that the cognitive capacities of patients are often diminished by the circumstances of their illness and hospitalization. Other studies have shown that patients often retain little of the information that is provided to them—a fact that practicing physicians have long known. (In one study, recordings were made of preoperative conversations between physicians and patients to establish a record of the informing process. Postoperative inquiries revealed substantial distortion and failures of memory when patients were asked to recall the conversations. One patient affirmed that he had been told nothing about his illness or the surgery that he faced, yet the recordings prove he had been provided with detailed information and an opportunity to raise questions and had reflected in his own conversation a good understanding of his medical circumstances.[1]) Finally, some medical procedures are so complicated or controversial that a layman can hardly be expected to have the necessary background information to understand what is really at issue in a decision about treatment.

Critics of the woman in the biopsy case held that it was foolish of her to think that she could make a better decision than her physicians about an issue so complicated that even the medical community was having difficulty deciding what the best course of treatment should be in cases like hers. Some physicians, summing up these barriers to patient understanding, have concluded that informed consent is impossible to achieve because patients are never actually well informed, and cannot be. "Are we to interrupt their illnesses," they ask, "in order to send them through medical school so that they can understand as we do what their problems and options are?''

The attempt to achieve patient understanding, moreover, incurs various costs. It is demanding of time; it requires the physician to draw on skills and sensitivities that have not typically been well developed in medical training; and, some critics have argued, it is dangerous to the health of the patients. The danger purportedly is of two kinds. Patients, because of their necessarily limited understanding, may make decisions that are detrimental to their own health. Also, there is a danger that patients will be directly harmed by the fears and anxieties induced by a more accurate understanding of the risks and discomforts they actually face. Informing patients in accordance with the doctrine requires that they come to understand the nature of their illness, the available choices of treatment, the risks and expected benefits of each choice, and the reasons for and against each of the options. But the list of risks is inexhaustible; not only can patients suffer ill effects from drugs, anesthesia, and surgical mishaps, they can be dropped off the cart coming back from the recovery room, and they can strangle themselves on their intravenous lines. Such outcomes are wildly improbable, but not impossible, and thus must be mentioned if *all* the risks must be mentioned. Any patient with the slightest inclination to timidity, and whose illness is not itself life-threatening, will shrink in horror from such a panoply of risks and may then flee from treatment that would provide benefit with no undue risk.

These criticisms of the doctrine of informed consent have some force but are partly confused. It is true that patients cannot achieve a perfect understanding of their medical circumstances and of the options for action that are available to their physicians. For that matter, neither can the physician achieve a perfect understanding; we have already considered this point in the chapter on medical mistakes. Still, in general, the patient will understand the medical aspects of the situation less well than the physician will. It is also true that some patients, given a reasonable understanding of their circumstances, will forget both the information and the fact that they once possessed it, and some patients will suffer heightened anxiety that may impede their treatment when they are informed about their circumstances. But what follows from these facts? Surely it does not follow that physicians may just do as they think best despite the wishes of the patients. That does not follow even in cases where the physician's judgment is clearly superior to that of the patient. First, the fact that the patient's knowledge will always be imperfect, and will often be inferior to the physician's, does not alter the fact that the patient has dominion over his or her own body, such that (except in an emergency or other circumstances of radically diminished capacity) treatment imposed without permission is abuse. Secondly, the fact that knowledge is *imperfect* does not imply that it is *inadequate* for the purpose at hand. Thirdly, the fact that a patient may, will, or does make the wrong decision about treatment does not entail that the patient lacks the right to make that decision. Fourthly, the fact that patients may misremember or entirely forget the information on which their decision, for better or ill, was made does not entail that the decision, when made, was uninformed or ill-informed. Consider each point in turn.

Those who emphasize the impossibility of imparting *complete* understanding to the patient leave physicians themselves on the uninformed side of the line. Those who emphasize that patients cannot be as informed as their physicians have a more reasonable position. Both groups seem to think the point that patient understanding is limited has a significance that it simply does not have, however. The right not to be assaulted is not conditional on the extent to which one understands the motivation of the assault; the right to make choices about the fate of one's body does not presuppose a good understanding of the consequences of the choices one makes.

John Stuart Mill believed that the strongest argument against paternalism is the utilitarian argument that no one else is likely to know better than a given individual what is best for that individual to choose. But he also believed that there is a positive value in the exercise of autonomous choice, so that it is better for a person to make a choice in his own behalf than for someone else to impose that same choice on him.[2] More recent writers have held that the strongest argument against paternalism is not based on considerations of utility—that is, of producing good consequences—but rests instead on the fact that paternalistic intervention in another person's affairs is, except under very special circumstances, a violation of that other person's rights.[3] One who rejects this position, arguing that it is allowable to intervene in another person's life so long as that intervention serves the interest of the other person, is thereby placing the Principle of Beneficence in a more fundamental position than the Principle of Autonomy. Yet respect for persons—for their liberty and their right to express their individuality by pursuing a freely chosen course of action—supports the Principle of Autonomy. One can argue that doing good is more important than respecting personal autonomy, and one can thereby judge paternalistic acts of intervention to be more easily justified than would the staunch defender of personal autonomy. And there is no conclusive argument against such a position. But the price one must pay for holding such a position is precisely a diminished level of respect for the liberty and independence that constitute the foundation on which the argument for autonomy rests and on which the case for democracy is ultimately based.

The point that patient knowledge is always imperfect, while true, has little force unless one also adds an argument that imperfect knowledge is inadequate to allow patients to make rational decisions about their treatment. The engineer's knowledge is imperfect, yet bridges are built, and most of them work. And the surgeon's knowledge is imperfect, yet surgery proceeds. So the question must be whether the knowledge that a patient can achieve is adequate to the purpose at hand, not whether it is total.

The question parallels an issue at the very foundations of democracy in a technological age, for it raises the conflict between entitlement and expertise. More and more social issues, such as the treatment of radioactive waste disposal, the control of biological research laboratories, or the defense of endangered species, raise questions that interest a broad public that must rely to some extent on the judgment of specialists in various technical areas to provide the information necessary for a decision to be made by the electorate or by representative bodies established by the electorate to serve the public interest. It is tempting at times, especially amidst the intricacies and idiocies of many a public debate, to escape from the diffuse entanglements of democratic processes to the far more efficient methods of technocracy, in which decisions requiring reliance on technical matters are made by those whose expertise gives them a privileged access to technical understanding. But wisely we resist the temptation. War, we affirm, is too important to be left to the generals; education, too important to be left entirely in the hands of the teachers; and government, too crucial to be in the hands of a cadre of professional politicians. The costs of democracy are high, and the processes of social decision making are cumbersome and erratic. But the values are higher still, provided that we retain a respect for the individuals whose interests social organization exists to serve.

Plato's views on political organization were totally at variance with this position; recognizing the fallibility of judgments made by members of the public, and hence by the public as a collective body (and possibly influenced by the public condemnation of his teacher, Socrates), he argued that power should be placed in the hands of an elite—the philosopher kings—whose expertise, developed only after decades of moral and technical preparation, could be relied upon to lead the populace on a path devoid of error.[4] But the notion of a benighted public's being led by an illuminated elite is the stuff of which totalitarianism is made, and it is a political philosophy that cannot survive in a climate of respect for persons.

So we struggle along, never fully satisified with the ways in which we make decisions that have a substantial dependence on technical expertise, confident only that although we may from time to time make a decision in error, no error will be greater than relinquishing our authority to make, in the last analysis, the decisions about social policy that will exert a major effect on public affairs. And as we proceed, we discover that surprisingly often we can learn enough of the technical material quickly enough to ground our decisions in a solid appreciation of what is at issue technically. When we do that, of course, we rapidly realize that the decision turns on more than just the technical questions. Thus, in assessing the likelihood of a failure of equipment at a nuclear power plant, we need to rely on the judgment of experts. But we can understand much of what they have to say, and we can then come to have an understanding of the level of safety that is most probably involved in the plant. But is that level of safety high enough to justify building the plant? That is not a question that the experts can answer; that is not a matter for technical expertise. It is a matter of the setting of social policy, in which we all share a comparable voice and a comparable interest. The closer we look, the less attractive technocracy seems.

The fact that technocracy is an undesirable approach to social policy decisions does not by itself tell us much about decisions involving the interactions between physicians and patients. It is merely suggestive of the point that a person's having a superior understanding of the technical details involved in a situation does not automatically mean he should be making the decisions. Let us look explicitly at the problem in the medical context.

Some patients, because of their own cognitive and psychological characteristics and the nature of their illness, can become well informed about their medical circumstances. (Norman Cousins's *Anatomy of an Illness*[5] documents the way he took over, in cooperation with his physicians, the management of a grave illness.) Other patients, in other circumstances, do not have and cannot be brought to have any reasonable understanding of their circumstances. So the extent to which the patient can be informed varies from not at all to comparably with the physician. Somewhere along that spectrum, patients have enough understanding of the medical aspects of their circumstances to exercise reasonable choice. Below that level, the case for paternalism builds; above it, the case for autonomy dominates. The situation is complicated by the fact that any patient's position on the spectrum of understanding is likely to depend on the quality of the physician's efforts to induce understanding in the patient. The better the physician is as an educator of the patient, the stronger the case is for respecting the autonomy of the patient. It becomes necessary, therefore, to make some assessment in the course of treatment—subject to revision at any point—of the extent to which the patient is, or can be made, capable of achieving a level of understanding that is adequate to support an autonomous choice.

Just as the decision about what to do in regard to a social policy involving technical issues will depend on more than the technical issues alone, medical decisions are often too important to be made on medical grounds alone. Consider again the woman who limited her consent to the biopsy procedure. Had the diagnosis been a finding of malignancy, many further technical questions about the nature of her disease and the possible modes of treatment would have arisen at once. The best source of knowledge about these matters is surely the medical profession and those in related areas. But nonmedical factors could also have an important bearing. If, for example, the woman were by profession and continuing aspiration a world-renowned nude model for painters and photographers, the prospect of a mastectomy might be even more distasteful than it ordinarily is. And that difference, at a given level of medical risk, might make the difference in what treatment the patient selects. Comparable considerations would apply to a man whose work as a model for bathing suit advertisements would be ended by the scarring that a coronary bypass operation would produce; he might on that account favor medical management of his angina, even if it seemed slightly less likely to be effective.

If it is assumed that the only rational option is the one with the best medical prognosis, then it follows trivially that a decision with a lower prospect of success is irrational. But there is no good reason to accept that assumption; there is no reason to believe that the prospect for medical success is the only relevant basis, or ought always to be the dominant basis, for exercising choice in medical situations. An individual has the right, in general, to determine what levels of risk to run in pursuit of the objectives that give his or her life its purpose and character; we recognize this in the case of dangerous occupations (the test pilot or high-wire artist, for example), dangerous recreations (hang gliding or American football), and dangerous life-styles (dietary imprudence or smoking). Why, then, should we suppose that just because one is in the role of patient, one's freedom to choose medically inferior options suddenly is dissipated?

The woman in our example might have assessed the comparative risks and decided to trade a small increment in prospects for medical success in exchange for avoiding a treatment destructive of her career. Whether or not such a choice makes sense for the patient is, in any case, not a medical question; it is a question that arises out of her medical circumstances and depends importantly on the medical facts, but it is a question the answer to which will depend in the final analysis on her values and priorities and to the place among them that she accords to matters of physical well-being, compared with vanity, accomplishment, competing demands on time and economic resources, and the like. The wrong decision from a purely medical point of view may thus not be the wrong decision from the broader perspective of the patient's life; the medical experts therefore have an important place in the decisions that must be made about treatment, but they have no basis for presuming to be able always to reach decisions about what, all things considered—medical and nonmedical alike—is best for the patient.

Lastly, it should be clear that the notion of the right decision is itself liable to be somewhat misleading, as if there were a single choice that is correct, with the challenge facing both physician and patient being that of identifying that one right choice, and the penalty for missing it being some sort of clear failure. A choice can be wrong if it aims at achieving certain objectives which it then fails to achieve; such is the case in the choice of an antibiotic to which the offending bacteria are resistant, and such is the case if a treatment selected to maximize survival leads instead to hastening death. But if a choice of treatment (or a refusal to be treated) leads to a life that is shorter, while at the same time allows for achieving more of the goals in one's plan of accomplishment, it is hard to see how that choice can properly be called wrong, even though there is a clear sense in which medical personnel, who can be expected to grant pride of place to medical considerations, might reasonably see it as the wrong choice. Further, if the choice is wrong not only medically but from the point of view of the patient's overall perspective as well, it still does not follow that it is necessarily wrong for the patient to have been allowed to make the choice, although it would be appropriate for medical personnel to try to help the patient understand how the choice fails to accord with the patient's overall values.

Just as a respect for freedom requires us to allow people to make choices in other dimensions of life—choices that can be described only as folly from any point of view—so, too, is the patient's right of choice undiminished by the possibility of failure in choosing. The right to choose is not limited to the right to choose rightly. Lack of understanding can, in any area of choice that affects us, lead to our making choices we will later regret; the wise among us will seek where we can find it the best available evidence on which to base the choices we make. But being uninformed does not in general reduce our rights of choice in matters that concern us solely; the right to choose is not generally limited to the right to choose knowledgeably either.

That this fact is often obscured in medical situations may be due to the assumption—usually justified—that a single goal is shared by the patient and the medical staff, that being to maximize the health of the patient. On that assumption, a choice that serves the goals of the medical staff is necessarily the choice that serves the best interests of the patient, and it seems only efficient to have the choice made on the basis of the most sophisticated understanding of the issues involved—that is, to have the choice made by the physician, who, in consultation with peers, is medically best informed. Even this, however, is an erroneous judgment; that a physician and patient share a common objective does not nullify the patient's rights of autonomous decision, even when the physician is clearly better informed than the patient about how to achieve the objective they share.

Those who have shown that patients often remember badly—and sometimes not at all—what they have been told about their medical conditions and treatment options have not shown that informed consent is impossible. They have simply reported research confirming a phenomenon about patient memory. Still, it is tempting to conclude, as some in medical practice surely do, that since patients in the end don't know the difference anyway, the responsible physician will—indeed, must—decide and do what is best for the patient. But making an informed decision does not assure remembering the basis of the decision at a later time—especially when subsequent events are of a highly stressful sort. Ask a friend or yourself, for that matter, why you chose the career you did, or the spouse you have, let alone the car you drive or the neighborhood you live in, and you will be reminded of the difficulty of being able, after the fact, to give a clear account of the reasons that led to decisions that constitute a major influence on the course of our lives. Often, in the making of such decisions, we were never clear about the reasons. But often, even where there was clarity, that clarity quickly fades with the passage of time. A patient who does not remember being informed about the nature of an illness or the decisions that had to be made about its treatment may nonetheless have been well informed at the time the decision was made. Such lapses of memory may create a problem from the point of view of the psychological well-being of the patient, however, and, correspondingly, place the physician in greater jeopardy.

A patient who does not remember being informed may be discontent at the thought of not having been informed, and the physician may be concerned about the consequences of that discontent for the patient's recovery, the physician's reputation, or even, in an extreme case, the physician's legal responsibility. So it may be necessary to become more careful about documenting that patients have been informed; relying on their recollections is obviously not enough. But there is no reason to assume that informing them better would change the situation, for there is no reason to assume that the cause of faulty memories of the informing transactions is that the informing was inadequately done. Compare here what anyone remembers about a subject on the way in to a final examination with what that same individual remembers about the subject even a few weeks later. Knowledge is a transient phenomenon for most people about most things.

Even one who agrees that informed consent is required by a proper respect for patient autonomy may still argue that the realities of clinical practice make the principle impossible to honor except in cases of unusual simplicity. The time and effort required to produce a high level of understanding by the typical patient are more than can reasonably be allocated by the typical physician without placing the fulfillment of other responsibilities in jeopardy, so moral *costs* are associated with informing patients fully. The physician who aspires to meet too high a standard as an educator of patients will have to sacrifice performance in some other dimension of practice; the result may be poorer-quality medical care or a more limited distribution of medical care, and these outcomes are morally more distressing than an imperfect regard for patient autonomy—especially since, as a matter of statistical likelihood, most patients do want treatment decisions to be made on the best possible medical grounds, do have a high degree of confidence in their own physicians—no matter how skeptical they may be about the medical profession as a whole—and are quite willing or even eager to be spared the rigors of learning and deciding about the medical choices that bear on their circumstances.

This argument, I think, has substantial force. But it does not tell against the claim that patients have a right to be informed about their medical circumstances and to make the choices that arise within those circumstances. Rather, it establishes the point that those rights are not the sole considerations, or even the sole morally significant considerations, that must be taken into account in the management of an illness. For instead of showing that patients cannot be properly informed, the argument rests on the fact that the costs of informing patients, like their capacity to achieve understanding, vary over a broad scale. At one end of the scale is the patient who can be easily and fully informed; at the other is the patient with diminished capacity who cannot achieve any reasonable level of understanding. Between lie a variety of cases requiring the physician to make an assessment both of the patient's capacity to achieve understanding and of the costs to the physician of inducing that level of understanding. Neither of these decisions is, in the traditional sense, a medical decision; neither is the sort for which physicians are typically trained in any explicit way. There is an assumption, and sometimes an expressed hope, that the skills and sensitivities required for such discrimination will be acquired through the processes of apprenticeship that constitute such a powerful part of medical training, but I see no basis for assuming that such hopes are sufficient.

The situation is further complicated by the fact that some patients can be harmed by the provision of information about their conditions. Consider the hypothetical patient Mr. Angstimmer. Hospitalized for a cardiac arrest, he is discovered in the course of examination to have a neurological disease of moderate severity. The disease is treatable with new drugs, but Mr. A. has a substantial and irrational fear of the disease, a more serious form of which ravaged two of his ancestors in earlier years. His prospects for recovery from the heart attack are good, but not yet excellent; he is still in intensive care and is agitated and anxious about his condition. Every effort is being made to keep him calm and to be as reassuring as possible without being deceptive. And then he asks a question that can be truthfully answered only by informing him about the discovery of the neurological problem—perhaps he asks about the nature or purpose of some medication he is asked to take. Under such conditions, it is reasonable or even obligatory to withhold the truth from the patient, on the ground that the risk of harm is so great as to override the demands of honesty and patient autonomy. The patient is weakened, both physically and psychologically, by his circumstances and is in the care of one whose primary responsibility is to protect and advance the interests of that patient insofar as they are directly connected with his health. (The heart attack may have been precipitated by the news that an investment had failed; it is nonetheless no responsibility of the physician to take over the management of the patient's investment portfolio—no matter how sophisticated the physician may be at investment management.) If the patient dies, his future autonomy is obliterated; the case for paternalistic management of the patient can thus itself be based on a respect for autonomy. To protect the patient's future freedom of action, we override his right to be informed in the present, constraining liberty in the interest of a larger liberty.[6] Importantly, this is done not by a stranger, but by one who bears a special responsibility for the care of the patient—just as the parent bears a special responsibility for the care of the child.

Indeed, some patients clearly prefer not to be as fully informed about their circumstances as their physicians might be inclined to make them. A number of physicians have reported to me having had patients complain on occasion that they were receiving more information than they wanted. If we wish to grant full respect to a patient's right to decide autonomously what is to be done to him or her physically, is there any good reason to refuse to allow the option of remaining in ignorance, trusting the physician to gather and use the relevant medical information in the ways that accord with the best medical judgment?[7] If we refuse to allow this choice, the requirement of informed consent then becomes not only a responsibility of the physician but an obligation of the patient, who must be informed even in the face of resistance to the imposition of the knowledge.

There are, of course, situations in which it is required that individuals receive certain kinds of information before they can proceed to the completion of transactions upon which they have embarked. Loans cannot be consummated until the borrower acknowledges being informed about the interest costs, one cannot ride a mule to the floor of the Grand Canyon without admitting to an understanding of the rigors involved and waiving the right to make claims against the management for falling victim to the associated risks, and so on. But in other situations we do not require enlightenment on the part of agents; one need not know anything about a car to buy it, a house to rent it, or even a child to have it. Sometimes, for the protection of the physician as much as that of the patient, it is required that a patient acknowledge an understanding of what is in store. In other circumstances, such as the case of Mr. Angstimmer, the patient is neither told nor allowed to learn what is in store. Yet we have no general clarity about how to distinguish cases of the first kind from cases of the second.

Further, there may be circumstances in which informing a patient can be damaging in subtler ways than those suggested by the case of Mr. Angstimmer. In his case the justification for not providing completely honest disclosure was the high risk that the information would increase the patient's anxiety to a point that directly threatened his cardiac stability and hence his life. But some have argued that informed consent can be damaging in less direct ways. The physician's therapeutic effectiveness rests in part upon the psychological power of the patient's trust in the benevolence and healing ability of the physician. There is some science in medical practice, but there is some magic as well. A physician's aura of confidence can have a calming influence on a patient, and a patient's trust can hasten recovery, even when that trust would be undermined by an understanding of just how uncertain the physician really is about the case. Yet trust can sometimes be increased by the knowledge that the physician is completely honest and will share his uncertainties with the patient. Too little is known about these phenomena beyond the fact that they are real and powerful.

Complicating the situation further is the fact that the physician is likely aware that clinical judgments are based on a mix of data of varying degrees of validity, combined with a good dose of hunch based on anecdotal experience, with a bit of outright guessing mixed in as well. The physician may be aware that some studies have shown a drug to be effective for a small majority of patients in a certain category, though other studies have been inconclusive. And the nature of the side effects may be in some dispute. Still, the physician had great success once using the drug on a patient who seemed similar in circumstances to the present patient. So perhaps it is worth a try, despite the physician's uncertainty about the reliability of the studies, the risk of side effects, and the relevance of the one successful case taken as a possible precedent. How much of the uncertainty that courses through the physician's head in such circumstances should be shared with the patient? If there is dispute in the medical literature about the drug, based on disagreement about the statistical significance of experimental results, should the physician involve the patient in a discussion of issues related to statistical significance? Or should the physician, in the interests of greater therapeutic effectiveness, pretend to less uncertainty than is actually present, while perhaps acknowledging that there is a certain amount of trial and error in medical practice?

The physician who has a conscientious concern with informing the patient is thus faced with at least these questions: (1) How much understanding can the patient achieve? (2) What is the patient's background information on which to build that understanding? (3) What will it cost in time and effort to achieve that understanding? (4) What are the psychological barriers to understanding? (5) Does the patient want the information? (6) What is the likelihood that the information will harm the patient either directly or by impeding the processes of recovery? (7) How much of what the patient could be made to understand is necessary for a reasonable level of informedness in the actual circumstances? (8) What portion of the information, if any, must the patient be made to understand independently of the patient's desire for information? (9) How much of

the physician's skepticism about the relevant information should be revealed to the patient? And, finally (10), when and how should the information be provided?

These questions are easy to answer in some cases but can be extremely
hard in other cases. Rarely are they addressed explicitly; rather, the
physician typically tends to respond to a case instinctively, relying on
the clinical judgment that is an amalgam of what has been learned from
previous successes and failures in practice and consultation with others
when a case seems particularly problematic.

Our focus has been on the informing side of the requirement of informed
consent; now consider the concept of consenting. On the way into the
operating room a surgeon once asked the surgical resident, "Did you get
the consent?"

"Yes, here it is," replied the resident, handing the surgeon a consent
form signed by the patient. But consent is not the sort of thing that one
can carry in one's pocket to an operating room and hand to a surgeon.
Just as numbers can be large or small, odd or even, but never heavy or
blue, consent can be reluctant, coerced, freely given, or denied, but never
carried around in a pocket. Consent is not a physical object; it is an act
of the will—and therefore not a piece of paper that is, at best, evidence
that the act took place. And evidence can be misleading. The reason it
is important not to confuse the signed consent form with the consent itself
is precisely that if one takes the signed form to be what is required, one
can adopt a far less stringent standard regarding consent than if one
remains aware that the consent requirement may not have been met even
in cases where the document gives evidence that it has been.

If I have reason to want you to undergo a treatment that you do not
want, I can produce a signed consent form by causing you to sign it under
duress. I may hold a gun to your head and threaten you with loss of life
if you do not sign. Or I may be your employer, who threatens you with
a loss of your job in the hazardous chemicals laboratory if you do not
agree to undergo a tubal ligation to eliminate any risk of a malformed
child resulting from your exposure to chemicals or to radiation in the lab.
In the case of the gun, no one could claim that an act of voluntary consent
had occurred; rather, it would be clear to all, once the facts were known,
that the signature on the consent form was obtained under duress, that
the evidence was therefore fraudulent, and that the requirement of informed consent had not been met. In the case of coercion by the employer,
the situation is less clear since the pressures brought to bear on the woman
are far less direct, and the choices less sharply drawn. Faced with the

choice of signing a consent form or being shot to death, most people in most circumstances would see themselves as having no choice—and therefore not acting freely. But the employee can refuse to accept the employer's terms. These are, he would argue, conditions that must be met only if she wishes to retain employment that she is free to give up. One's life circumstances may be such that the loss of a job would be devastating, however, and hence a case that undue coercion has been brought to bear can be made in such situations.

Again, the consent form provides definitive evidence only of a physical act—the signing. In the normal course of events one assumes that the physical act of signing a consent form will occur only as a consequence of a cognitive act of agreement having taken place. And as a matter of statistical likelihood, the assumption may be well warranted. But it is not always true. The physician whose responsibility it is to gain consent thus has a responsibility to distinguish between a form bearing a signature and an act of consent. That requires understanding the *process* by which the form came to be signed and considering that process in awareness of all the ways such a process can go wrong.

Some have argued that consent is never freely given in the context of medical treatment because illness, medication, fear of death, and pain add up to a coercion as powerful as the gun. But even if this observation accurately describes some situations, it does not seem to cover many others, where the distortions of consciousness that can accompany illness may be wholly lacking. A subtler and more serious argument rests on the implicitly coercive power of the physician's role: Patients will do what their physicians want them to do, if for no other reason than because of fear—fear of a bad medical outcome and fear of the consequences of defying the wishes, however subtly they are expressed, of the physician. But this is a hard argument to make plausible to physicians, who have to deal with the problems of compliance that arise when patients openly reject, or simply ignore, clear and direct indications of what their physicians take to be medically advisable or even necessary. Yet the argument has some force, for physicians do communicate by subtle cues as well as by overt expression, and they can sometimes influence their patients more than they realize. A change in tone of voice or facial expression, while describing treatment options, can betray a preference that tacitly pressures the patient into consenting as the physician would wish. In the relationship between physician and patient, the differential of power is so massive that the patient may be unable to resist seeing the physician as providing only one real option. The physician, so the argument goes, must be meticulous in an effort to provide information in a neutral way that does not pressure the patient to choose one way or another because of the physician's preferences.

This argument, were it good, would entail that a patient's physician, who is most likely the best-informed of anyone involved in the case, should be effectively barred from rendering advice of a medical sort— precisely the one sort of advice to which the physician can lay claim as an expert. We need not embrace such a bizarre outcome to be mindful of the problem of undue physician influence. There is nothing inappropriate about medical advice's being the dominant factor in decisions about medical treatment so long as the process of decision retains a place for the incorporation of other values that may be in conflict with a single-minded pursuit of medical objectives. If a physician is aware of the distinction between medical factors and those nonmedical factors that can play a role in the making of a medical decision, and if the physician is sensitive to the ways in which consent can be coerced, there should be no objection to the physician's expressing a preference explicitly about what would be medically best for the patient to do. The patient may not resist the force of that preference, but what is most important is that the circumstances allow for the possibility of such resistance.

The physician who has a conscientious concern with the patient's consent is thus faced with this additional question: (11) Is the consent voluntary, or is it the result of coercion or undue influence?

These eleven questions pose a challenge to the most conscientious physician. At the same time, they underscore the extent to which therapeutic transactions depend on an effective relationship between physician and patient. The more the patient understands, and the more the patient is willing and able to assume a share of the responsibility of entering into a collegial relationship with the physician in the management of medical care, the greater the likelihood that they will be able to join forces effectively in pursuit of shared objectives. In fact, patients are often sadly unable to accept such responsibility, and physicians are left to grapple with the problems of informed consent and autonomy with little help from those in their care. How well prepared are they to meet this challenge? Is this sort of expertise provided by the training they receive?

4

Illness, Life,
and the Good Patient

"When you've got your health," preaches the lady in a television commercial, "you've got just about everything." Yet many people behave as if they do not take their health very seriously; they pursue other objectives than physical well-being even at substantial cost to their health. Their critics admonish them to reform, often claiming that they owe it to themselves to take better care of themselves, that health is something one has an obligation to pursue or maintain. The value of health, commonly assumed, is rarely argued for, however. We are left with the oddity of a general belief that health is good and illness bad, conjoined with widespread behavior that is medically imprudent or even reckless. I want to explore this phenomenon, asking whether one does in fact have an obligation to attend to one's health, examining the reasons why illness is bad, and probing the basis of the conviction that life itself is of great value. Then I will draw some conclusions for the way patients ought to be treated and the way they ought to behave.

There are cases—the woman seeking an abortion for nonmedical reasons, the chronic overeater, the smoker, the alcoholic or other drug addict, the discontented homosexual, the person seeking plastic surgery to obscure the manifestations of advancing age for reasons of vanity, the child abuser—where we may be uncertain about whether we are dealing with illness or with phenomena of other sorts, and we may be uncertain about whether to classify such people as patients even when they seek medical responses to their situations. But I will set such issues aside and here consider only clear cases, such as the person hospitalized for treatment of what is uncontroversially accepted as a medical problem or otherwise seeking medical help for an uncontroversial physical ailment. (Of course, not all patients are ill, not all sufferers from illness are patients, and not all victims of disease are sufferers at all.)

Is it correct to speak of health as something one has a duty to pursue or maintain? Do people who act in ways detrimental to their health not only act imprudently but also violate some moral obligation? If there is an obligation in regard to health, to whom is it an obligation, and what is its origin? Consider first some general characteristics of obligations or duties.

Every obligation is an obligation to act in some specifiable way. For example, an obligation to be a person of honest or charitable character is an obligation to act in honest or charitable ways. To be under an obligation to perform some action means that at least on the face of it, one is morally culpable if one does not do it. It can be justifiable to violate an obligation, but one must have a good reason. If I promise to meet you promptly at five, I am under an obligation to do so. But violation of that obligation is justified if I have stopped to save a drowning child. Even then I owe you at least an explanation. Of course, if I had been able to telephone you, you could have released me from my obligation. That obligation gave you certain rights in regard to my behavior, but you were free to waive those rights.

Obligations can arise from promises, contracts, agreements, and even implicit understandings. Such obligations—called special obligations— involve an agent who is under the obligation, someone to whom the agent is obligated, and some action. Special obligations thus have this general form: One person is obligated to another to perform some action. If he wishes to do so, the second person may release the first person from the obligation; otherwise, the first person owes the second person either the action or an acceptable justification for nonperformance—the second person has a right to these things.

The action may benefit the second person, as when I have an obligation to pay you an agreed amount for the rental of your house. The action may benefit some third party, as when I have an obligation to care for your child because I am under contract with you to do so. Or the action may be to the agent's own benefit, as when you promise your friend that you will take a much-needed vacation. Actions of this last kind, which benefit the agent who performs them, are called self-regarding. There can be various reasons for performing self-regarding actions, including an obligation to someone else to do so.

Does it make sense to speak of obligations to *oneself*, as in "You owe it to yourself to stop smoking so much"? One interpretation of such admonitions is that if you do not change your ways, you will be acting contrary to your own best interests—your aspirations and objectives will be impeded by your imprudence. On this interpretation the admonition is sound advice, but not *moral* advice. It would be imprudent not to reform, but the claim does not have the force of the claim, for example, that you ought to act kindly toward those who are suffering or pay to another what you owe. Is there a moral sense in which you owe it to yourself to be prudent?

Immanuel Kant held that duties to oneself—to preserve one's life, maintain one's health, and develop one's talent—were the most central of obligations.[1] But it is hard to make sense of the notion of an obligation to oneself. For an obligation from which one can release oneself at will has no binding force. Yet if you are the person to whom you are purportedly obligated, then you, because you hold the rights that follow from the obligation, can simply waive those rights and release yourself from the obligation. So an obligation to preserve or enhance one's own health apparently cannot be an obligation *to* oneself, even though such an obligation would be self-regarding.

It might still be that one has an obligation to oneself in regard to one's health—if it can be shown that there are obligations, unlike the special obligations we have been discussing, that do not arise from any sort of promise, contract, or agreement and are not subject to nullification by those who gain rights because of them. This was Kant's position; he argued that pure reason, independently of any actions performed by people or relationships among them, was the source of moral obligations—including obligations in regard to one's own health and life. Unless one is willing to adopt some such position, however, it does not seem likely that one can defend the idea of obligations to oneself.

The statement that one owes it to oneself to try to be healthy need not be taken as simple nonsense, however. Rather, it can be taken as a prudential maxim of unusually broad applicability. For whatever one's aspirations and objectives, whatever one's conception of the good life, it is highly likely that one's interests will be advanced by health and impeded by illness. One owes it to oneself to be healthy, then, in the sense that one is usually foolish from the point of view of one's present and future desires if one acts so as to undermine one's health. But this is not by itself a moral point. It may be unfortunate in many ways for one to be very foolish, but it is not necessarily a violation of any obligation.

Even if one cannot literally be obligated to oneself to try to be healthy, one *can* have explicit obligations to others that require one to protect and defend one's health. Athletes, astronauts, and others for whom excellence of physical condition is a prerequisite for professional success could be contractually bound to act prudently in respect to their health. In such cases the obligation to be healthy would be an explicit duty, requiring the individual, under threat of legal as well as moral culpability, to act prudently in regard to health. But the obligation to be healthy can have other origins also. If I am obligated to you to do something, then I am obligated to do whatever else is necessary for the doing of it. For example, if I owe you a home-cooked dinner, I am also obligated to obtain the ingredients. If I default, I cannot escape blame simply on the ground that I neither had nor tried to get the food. So the obligation to get the food is derivative from the obligation to cook the dinner. Are there obligations unrelated to health that have derivative obligations that do require regard for one's health?

Some obligations have nothing to do with health. If I undertake to provide financially for the education of your children, I can fulfill the obligation through trusts or insurance so that I avoid becoming obligated to perform any self-regarding actions. But other obligations do require the maintenance of one's health. If you promise to be my traveling companion for the summer, I have a right to expect you to try to maintain a state of health that is compatible with travel. If you default because of illness induced by reckless behavior against sound medical advice, I can justly claim to have been let down in a morally culpable way.

Certain special relationships involve the undertaking of special obligations, such as those incurred in marriage, which bind the participants to each other in certain legally specified ways. But beyond these specified obligations there exist further obligations implicit in that special relationship—obligations that reflect the individual characteristics of the particular pattern of expectations and interdependencies that have nurtured the relationship. To enter into a marriage, at least of anything like the traditional sort, is to undertake voluntarily to pursue and sustain a pattern of interaction that typically will require the maintenance of one's health. Illness usually befalls its victims through no culpable behavior on their part, but illness is sometimes invited or induced by negligent or reckless behavior. In some cases it can make sense to blame someone for being ill precisely because that illness results from the violation not merely of prudential maxims but of moral obligations as well.

Similar arguments apply to the maintenance of life itself. No one has a special obligation to himself, literally speaking, to preserve his life. But one can have obligations to others the fulfillment of which is incompatible with one's death. Thus, close relatives of someone who commits suicide feel anger and resentment, along with their remorse and guilt, not only commonly but justifiably, when the suicide leaves obligations unfulfilled.

As we have seen, some writers, such as Kant, argue that obligations that require the maintenance of one's health exist independently of the special relationships one has to others. But one need not embrace Kant's theories to believe that there are obligations that transcend the specific actions and special relationships of mankind. For example, one who accepts a theologically based conception of moral obligations might argue that obligations in regard to one's health have a divine origin. John Locke held that one's life is a property over which one has no jurisdiction; rather, it is held in trust, being of divine ownership—in consequence, one has obligations to preserve and protect it.[2] Or it might be argued that one's status as a member of the human community itself imparts obligations of a variety of sorts—obligations to one's fellowman—such as the obligation to be charitable to those in need or the obligation to refrain from gratuitous assault. If such general obligations do exist, some of them may have as consequences other obligations that are self-regarding.

Even apart from such entirely general obligations, however, one can be in circumstances that make plausible the presence of moral obligations that arise independently of one's contracts, agreements, or familial relationships. Imagine an isolated, shipwrecked society with just one physician. One might well argue that the physician is under an obligation to provide for future medical care as he approaches advancing age—that he *ought* to take an apprentice and pass on his skills for the sake of his survivors and future generations. And one might well mean not merely that it would be socially desirable for the physician to do so but that he is morally culpable if he refuses. Nor does there seem to be anyone in a position to release him from such an obligation. His acceptance of the apprentice, moreover, might entail further self-regarding obligations, at least until the apprentice is trained well.

Of course, even when a self-regarding obligation in respect to health does exist, that obligation cannot, strictly speaking, be to *be* healthy, for health is often beyond one's capacity to achieve or maintain. The obligation can at most be to take reasonable actions conducive to the state of health that is required by the other obligation one has. Without such other obligations, one would have no obligation to pursue health. People who are alone—devoid of relationships that bind them to others—may also be devoid of the aspirations that bind them to the future. Such tragic figures may lack the desire to maintain their health or even their lives, and there is no persuasive basis for arguing that they have any obligation to do so. Further, we can imagine circumstances under which the pursuit of health might be less tragically shunned. For example, a physician might wish to endure a temporary but moderately serious illness in order to experience directly the plight of the seriously ill—with a view toward enhancing his or her future ability to deal sensitively with patients. Or a writer, aspiring to produce a compelling portrayal of illness, might willingly embrace an ailment and forgo or defer medical care in the service of his art. It is hard to see how either could reasonably be accused of thereby violating any moral obligation, in the absence of other considerations.

Health, then, is an almost universally valuable state. Yet many are imprudent in the extreme in regard to their own health largely because they are motivated by other interests more strongly than by their concern to be well. It would be hard to argue convincingly that one literally owes it to oneself to be protective of one's health, no matter how desirable health is acknowledged to be. But most owe it to others, for a variety of reasons, to seek and maintain good health. Those who lack any such obligation are free to abandon their health and even their lives without thereby violating a moral obligation. But that freedom exists only in consequence of the chilling impoverishment of their lives.

If one grants that health is desired by people to a degree which, while it may not dominate their decisions, at least typically constrains them, it seems clear that illness is an evil to be avoided. There are, of course, situations in which people derive positive benefits from illness. It can exempt them from discomforting responsibilities, gain them the concern and attention of others by whom they feel too little regarded, and in various additional ways provide secondary gains that can even cause some people to nurture their illnesses and resist efforts aimed at curing them. Still, for most people, most of the time, illness is judged to be undesirable, and the prospect of recovery is welcomed.

It is worth clarifying just what it is about illness that makes it undesirable because the way in which one responds to illness will depend not simply on the fairly crude judgment that illness is bad but on the particular respects in which it is judged to be bad. The two most obvious concomitants of illness that cause it to be viewed with disfavor are discomfort and dysfunction. When we feel ill—whether the feeling is of mild distress or acute pain—we naturally want to feel better, if for no other reason than to replace unpleasant feelings with pleasant ones. And when we are incapacitated, we are unable to pursue our objectives—be they modest or grand—and the frustration and loss of progress yield a kind of psychic pain that can also be acute. These two features of illness are well understood, and rarely forgotten, by the medical profession. But they are not the only features of illness that make it distasteful.

If an illness is serious enough to involve significant discomfort or disability, it tends also to command center stage in the consciousness of its victim. The result is a kind of egocentricity—an absorption in one's own physical circumstances—that shrinks the world of one's concerns and thereby diminishes one. Further, the patient can be well aware of this diminution and can find the egocentricity from which there is no obvious escape to be a source of crushing boredom. That is not the only reason that sickness is so boring, of course; that one may be constrained with respect to location, diet, exertion, and the like also contributes. But the egocentricity can be an additional source of boredom, especially as the patient comes to fear that it is sure to be boring to others. The dependency that accompanies serious illness also contributes to the diminution of the patient's self-image. And finally, illnesses of a nontrivial sort, even if they are nowhere close to being life-threatening, can be patient-threatening in their implicit affirmation of human mortality. The hospital setting, which offers most inpatients at least an occasional glimpse of patients in far worse condition, helps underscore the point.

Many of these factors—the boredom of illness, the egocentricity it promotes, the discomforting fear of death it may prompt, the dependency it induces, and the diminution of self-image that results—may have little bearing on the patient's prospects for recovery. If the physician's concern is to *eliminate* the illness, thereby to eliminate the pain and dysfunction it brings, these factors may be of little interest. Only insofar as they may be an impediment to cure need they be considered. But if the physician's objective is to *see the patient through* the illness, as opposed to getting the patient past the illness, these factors assume a larger importance. Quite apart from the eventual outcome of a medical case, the quality of the experience of the illness can depend greatly on the extent to which the treatment of that illness, and the overall handling of the patient during the period of treatment, take these factors into account.

One source of disagreement about how medical care should proceed arises from different degrees of concern with the process of treatment and how it is experienced, on the one hand, and the outcome of treatment, on the other. Thus, the radiologist who is single-mindedly concerned with taking good pictures and reading them flawlessly may be utterly insensitive to the humiliation and even rage that may be felt by his patients as they are ignored at length, then shuffled shivering from one delay to another before their turn on the table comes up. The patient who complains disrupts the system of care, taking time, causing distraction, and sometimes offending medical support personnel, who prefer it to be a matter of trust that the handling of patients is being conducted in the best way. Such a complainer may come to be viewed as not being a good patient. But what is it to be a good patient, after all?

In one sense of the phrase, the answer is easy. A good patient is one who places the value of recovery above all, follows directions, offers information appropriately, places no excessive demands on medical staff, and has a pleasant disposition as well. Such a patient is easiest to manage and hence will be expected to recover as quickly and completely as possible. This idealized patient *is* good from the perspective of health care personnel faced with the responsibilities of patient management. They can be forgiven their preference for such patients if we remember that patients are sometimes deceptive, uncooperative, demanding, and nasty. But there is another perspective—that of the patient. What is it, from a patient's point of view, that makes a good patient?

A woman was recovering from major surgery. Although strong narcotics were available on request every three or four hours, she had virtually given them up. Her tolerance for pain was fairly high, and she strongly disliked the diminution of alertness that the analgesics cause. Her intravenous lines had been infiltrating repeatedly, however, and one arm was sore, swollen, and red in reaction to intravenous tetracycline.* A nurse was struggling to install a new IV line but could find only veins that were sorely bruised or collapsed. As she fished around with the needle in search of success, the patient's endurance came to an end. She began to cry and to complain. The nurse then patted her on the sorest part of the swollen arm and said, "There, there, dear. Try to control yourself. I know it's uncomfortable."

The tears vanished. The patient turned to her husband and calmly said, " 'Uncomfortable.' This woman is mad. Get her out of here." He evicted the nurse and called for a resident physician. A short time later she arrived and deftly installed a new line. (It was not the medical degree that made the difference here; often the nurses are best at this procedure.) Perhaps thirty minutes later the patient rested comfortably—one eye half-opened in the direction of the television set. The nurse who had been ejected entered, carrying a syringe. The husband asked her, as he did anyone who entered the room, what she was carrying and with what intentions she came in.

"It's Valium," she replied. "It will help her relax."

"There is no order for Valium," he replied.

---

*An intravenous line is said to infiltrate when the IV needle punctures the wall of the vein, causing the nutrient fluid to collect in the surrounding tissue instead of entering the bloodstream.

"There is now," came her rejoinder. She had called the physician in charge of the case, reported an uncooperative or hysterical or overanxious patient, and been given authorization to administer a tranquilizer. The patient, nearly asleep when the nurse came in, said, "I am quite relaxed, and I will not take any Valium. I suggest you leave and consider giving it to yourself." The nurse withdrew.

In the nurse's judgment, the patient had taken an unfortunate turn and was no longer being a good patient. The situation called for psycho-pharmaceutical intervention. But from the patient's perspective, the situation was quite different. In her own eyes she was simply advocating her interests vigorously where they were being submerged amidst the complex demands of providing medical care. Her desire to be cooperative and uncomplaining was tempered by a concern with the processes of treatment and with a continuing sense of her right to act autonomously in her own behalf. And she was centrally concerned to maintain her right to express negative emotions, to respond honestly to distressing situations despite the discomfort that negative emotion might impose on the hospital staff.

Both patient and health care provider may agree that the overall objective is recovery and discharge of the patient, but along the way conflicts can arise at any point between the demands on providers and the shorter-term interests of the patient. The patient who is good in the sense of being good at the task, effective at making the best of the situation as judged from the perspective of that patient, is one who can competently advocate and protect his or her own interests; both where they coincide with those of the medical team and where they diverge or conflict.

The point is particularly well captured in Brian Clark's provocative drama *Whose Life Is It Anyway?*[3] Ken Harrison, a young sculptor who has been paralyzed from the neck down in a road accident, knows that his plight is permanent, and contemplates his fate with some distress. His physician, Dr. Scott, stops by the sister's (nurse's) office:

DR. SCOTT: Did you get that Valium for Mr. Harrison, Sister?
SISTER: Yes, Doctor. I was going to give him the first at twelve o'clock.
DR. SCOTT: Give him one now, will you?
SISTER: Right.
DR. SCOTT: Thank you . . . On second thoughts . . . give it to me. I'll take it. I want to talk with him.
SISTER: Here it is.
DR. SCOTT: Thank you. I've brought something to help you.
KEN: My God, they've got some highly qualified nurses here.
DR. SCOTT: Only the best in this hospital.
KEN: You're spoiling me you know, Doctor. If this goes on I shall demand that my next enema is performed by no one less than the Matron.

DR. SCOTT: Well, it wouldn't be the first she'd done, or the thousandth, either.

KEN: She worked up through the ranks, did she?

DR. SCOTT: They all do.

KEN: Yes, in training school they probably learn that at the bottom of every bed pan lies a potential Matron. Just now, for one or two glorious minutes, I felt like a human being again.

DR. SCOTT: Good.

KEN: And now you're going to spoil it.

DR. SCOTT: How?

KEN: By tranquilizing yourself.

DR. SCOTT: Me?

KEN: Oh, I shall get the tablet, but it's you that needs the tranquilizing; I don't.

DR. SCOTT: Dr. Emerson and I thought . . .

KEN: You both watched me disturbed, worried even perhaps, and you can't do anything for me—nothing that really matters. I'm paralyzed and you're impotent. This disturbs you because you're a sympathetic person and as someone dedicated to an active sympathy doing something—anything even— you find it hard to accept you're impotent. The only thing you can do is to stop me thinking about it—that is—stop me disturbing you. So I get the tablet and you get the tranquility.

DR. SCOTT: That's a tough diagnosis.

KEN: Is it so far from the truth?

DR. SCOTT: There may be an element of truth in it, but it's not the whole story.

KEN: I don't suppose it is.

DR. SCOTT: After all, there's no point in worrying unduly—you know the facts. It's no use banging your head against a wall.

KEN: If the only feeling I have is in my head and I want to feel, I might choose to bang it against a wall.

DR. SCOTT: And if you damage your head?

KEN: You mean go bonkers.

DR. SCOTT: Yes.

KEN: Then that would be the final catastrophe, but I'm not bonkers—yet. My consciousness is the only thing I have and I must claim the right to use it and, as far as possible, act on conclusions I may come to.

DR. SCOTT: Of course.

KEN: Good. Then you eat that tablet if you want tranquility, because I'm not going to.

DR. SCOTT: It is prescribed.

KEN: Oh come off it, Doctor. I know everyone around here acts as though those little bits of paper have just been handed down from Sinai. But the writing on those tablets isn't in Hebrew . . .

Of course, not all patients can advocate their own interests so articu-lately. Our son was hospitalized for a day when he was an infant. He was admitted late in the afternoon, as various shifts were changing. By seven he was fussing for food; upon inquiring, we were told that he had come in too late to get on the list for dinner, which in any case was no longer available. He didn't eat much in those days, but what little he ate meant a lot to him. The nursing supervisor couldn't help except to call for the resident. He saw no easy solution at first but in the end found a modest meal, appropriate for a hungry one-year-old, easier to provide than the home telephone number of the hospital director. During this negotiation a laboratory technician took a blood sample; this must surely be an odd event in the life of one too young to be given an explanation. A second technician later tried to do the same but agreed under pressure to check with the lab first; the order was a duplicate, and the assault was averted.

The infant is a pure case of a patient who has no defense against his medical care. If nothing went wrong in medical treatment, defense would not be an issue. But medical treatment is laced through with errors large and small, and it is thus important to consider how the necessary defenses can be achieved. In the case of an infant there must be some continuing presence, preferably independent of the medical team, to exercise surveillance and to advocate the interests of the patient; parents typically play this role. Had we not been present, our son would have gone without dinner and had an unnecessary blood sample taken; these are fairly small issues, and he would in all likelihood have been discharged just as quickly in any event—but with a somewhat less benign impression of the experience. And we *had* been advised to keep him calm—a state not encouraged by dietary deprivation or gratuitous bloodletting.

But the point does not depend on the minor perils avoided in this case, for serious perils too are sometimes avoided by vigilant protection of the interests of patients. There is no suggestion here that medical staffs are incompetent, unsympathetic, or ill-motivated. The problem arises primarily because medical care has become exceedingly complex and is now provided largely through institutional mechanisms that exhibit to varying degrees all the problems inherent in large bureaucracies of any sort. It is not just a question of physicians and nurses, but of appointment secretaries, bookkeepers, and aides, assistants, and apprentices of every stripe—all of whom can impinge on the lives of hospitalized patients, and remarkably many of whom can impinge on the lives of outpatients. Keeping them all properly coordinated so that they impinge on the patient in a consistent and helpful way requires a synoptic overview of the pattern of their interactions with the patient. But typically, the only person in a position to obtain such an overview is the patient. And the more seriously ill the patient is, the greater is the need for such advocacy. Yet the more seriously ill the patient is, the less able the patient is to play that role; indeed, the more seriously ill the patient is, the more the patient is like the infant, who must rely solely on others.

The possibility of a patient's exercising independent judgment is therefore reduced by the patient's medical circumstances to varying degrees; and others must sometimes fill the gap. There is a procedural simplicity to vesting in the physician the authority to make decisions whenever questions arise in regard to the handling of a patient, but that approach has a built-in flaw: It provides no safeguard to protect the interests of the patient when the values of the patient differ from those held explicitly or unwittingly by the physician. Further, it provides no answer to the problem of integrating the full array of medical services, including those of the physician, into a coherent approach. In principle, this problem need not arise, according to the received view of how medical services are to be coordinated. The physician coordinates and oversees all the services and conditions affecting the patient, keeping informed and maintaining control through the mechanism of the patient's medical record. But in fact, the record becomes one more variable in the system of services; it can contain errors, can be misread, can be maintained incompletely, and—especially since it is typically kept from the patient's view—can become an instrument in the management of the patient that does not reflect the values of the patient where they do diverge from those of the surrounding context of health care.

Finally, there is a distortion in the process that has its analogue in academic life. Professors easily can, and often do, overestimate their importance as influences on their students. What we do does make a difference, or at least can, but the total effect of a university experience for a student will depend as much on the other students, the general ambiance of the institution, and the unfolding of events in the world as on the actions of the faculty. Wise educators know this and try to keep the larger educational context in view when making decisions about the basic academic business of courses and curriculum. Similarly, physicians can underestimate the importance for patient welfare of the nonmedical factors in the patient's health care environment—such factors as hospital noise level, compatibility of roommates, ease of obtaining desired information, and even the decor. Wise physicians know this and try in their medical decision making to keep the larger context in view. But just as professors are typically entirely untrained in most matters that influence how they affect their students—the traditional, though false, presumption being that expertise in the discipline is all that is needed—physicians, too, can be utterly naïve outside the confines of their specialties and, as a result, can fail to understand the full range of factors influencing the course of a medical case.

Some medical cases present a moral dilemma plain for all to see. The famous Karen Quinlan case is of this kind; the question of whether or not it was morally justifiable to disconnect the respirator was a question of values that no physician or jurist claimed as falling cleanly within his field of expertise. Other cases involve moral dilemma less visibly. I would include here the problem of how much responsibility a physician bears to educate a patient and to protect the autonomy of that patient when the patient's illness or intellect produce barriers to efficient communication. A third class of cases includes those that do not involve any moral dilemma in the sense of presenting a difficult moral decision but that nonetheless have significant moral content in that there is a conflict of values importantly involved in the case. The case of the philosopher's mother is of this kind; the conflict was between the values implicitly assumed by the physician and those that were more closely linked to the patient's interests. The problem in cases of this sort is not so much to figure out the right thing to do as to ensure that the right thing gets done. For whenever decisions made in behalf of a patient reflect values that are not shared by the patient, there is a *prima facie* case that the autonomy of the patient has been overridden in an unwarranted way. This is especially so in cases where the patient could have made a decision independently but was not accorded the chance. It is less clear in those cases where the values of the patient are obscured by diminished capacity.

In cases of all these kinds, moral difficulty, when it arises, transcends the physician's scope of expertise; otherwise, the case would at worst be medically hard, not morally difficult. So, in any morally troubling case, there arises the question of who should bear the burdens of facing the moral problem and making the necessary decisions.

This question brings us to another classification of cases that cuts across the last one. In some cases patients are well able to make decisions in their own behalf and should be accorded the opportunity; this is exemplified by the woman hospitalized for a biopsy. In other cases some representative or advocate of the patient is in the best position to make decisions; this is exemplified by the philosopher whose mother was dying. But in some cases the physician must decide simply because no other mechanism of choice is available. This can be the case in emergency situations, in surgery, in neonatal crises. It is in just such situations that the physician is most in jeopardy of being accused of playing God, yet in such situations the physician may be acutely aware of the lack of any well-informed basis for making a moral choice about the life of another.

The physician may bear the burden with a sense of humility and out of a sense of responsibility to face alone the tasks for which there is no help. On other occasions there is help, however, as when those charged with responsibility for handling a case have recourse to the courts, advisory committees, or other broader mechanisms of decision.

It may be useful here to reflect on some general characteristics of making a decision. To decide is to choose among alternative actions. Competent decision making involves an assessment of all the available alternatives; people often make poor or even disastrous decisions simply because they neglect to consider all the possibilities. A decision need not involve any positive action; to refrain from making a decision is not necessarily to avoid making it. Rather, it is often to make the decision in a particularly shabby way, as when the patient dies while the medical staff is trying to decide whether or not to try to save him. When a decision is yours, deciding not to make it also is futile; that itself can produce one of the outcomes among which you were struggling to decide.

Jean-Paul Sartre, the late French existentialist, has some observations on this point.[4] He describes a young man in the French underground who deliberates about whether to flee France, abandon his dependent mother, and join the forces of liberation or to stay and work with the underground resistance movement. What is he to do? The man can seek the advice of a priest but must choose a resistance priest or a collaborationist priest. Given advice, he must still decide whether or not to follow that advice; anyone who tries to dispense with the need to make a decision by getting advice must ultimately accept the advice or reject it and thereby makes the decision in the end after all. It is Sartre's view that people are free to make decisions to a much greater extent than they realize and, when in a position to make a decision, cannot avoid doing so. Thus, we often hear someone say, "I wish I could," and then describe some course of action that we know perfectly well is possible, but that has just not been given a high enough priority to be chosen.

Sartre emphasizes that not only can we choose over a much wider range of options than we commonly realize, but we also reaffirm our decisions constantly by the choices we make. Every time one goes to work, one reaffirms the decision to be working; one could have stayed home, one could walk out at any moment. One facet of the medical decision-making problem is illuminated here. If one is in a position to influence a decision, what one does will influence the decision even if one would wish it otherwise. This is one reason why it is an error to rail against physicians for making decisions that present circumstances call on them to make. They sometimes decide badly, sometimes well, some-

times in pain and humility, and sometimes with an arrogant moral im-
perialism, but typically because the structure of health care delivery tends
to place them on the decisive spot. If we are discontent with the way the
decisions are sometimes made, we are better advised to consider the way
physicians are trained to bear the resultant burdens than simply to lament
what sometimes seem to be overarching medical prerogatives.

Let us review some of the ground we have just been over. Health is
not the only thing we value, nor do we owe it to ourselves in any literal
sense to pursue it. Most of us care a great deal about it, however, and
have relationships with others that require us to sustain that concern.
Medical staffs, quite reasonably, tend in the treatment of a patient to
place the highest priority on medical success as they interpret it; a potential
for conflict of values results. For health is ill-defined, and the patient's
objectives, even when health is placed above all, may not coincide with
those of the medical staff. (Which would count as better health for the
philosopher's mother, a longer but less comfortable life or a shorter but
more comfortable one?) Because the values of patients and of their physicians can differ, and especially in light of the complexity of contemporary
medical care and the prospects for errors of various sorts within the
systems of health care delivery, patients need some sort of effective
protection and advocacy of their interests. This need is compounded by
the fact that patients and physicians may differ in assessing the relative
importance of outcome and process in medical treatment. But patients
are often in no position to advocate their own interests effectively; their
capacity may be diminished—temporarily or permanently—so that they
cannot exercise informed and autonomous decisions in their own behalf.
The physician is typically in the best position to fill the gap because of
a privileged access to the relevant information, a greater level of understanding of it, and a position of authority that yields efficiency in the
implementation of decisions. Yet there are dangers inherent in the physician's powers, which can impose values on a patient that are not shared
by the patient. Making such decisions, well or badly, is unavoidable for
physicians under present circumstances; it is therefore worth considering
the prospects for enhancing the physician's ability to make them well.

A woman's husband had been dying of cancer for several months. He
had lingered on the brink of death for weeks. The same sort of sophisticated medical treatment that prolonged the dying of Franco and of Tito
so dramatically was also available to benefit him, even though he was
no head of state. His wife was worn to a point beyond hope, beyond

despair, beyond grief by the long and agonized dying. On a Friday afternoon, as she expressed a sense of futility to her husband's physician, he said, "Don't give up, Mrs. X. I think we can hold him through the weekend." The devastated woman snapped out of her torpor, fired the physician, and replaced him with one who made no effort to extend the life of the husband but instead helped him ease into death within the day.

All parties to this episode would agree that life is valuable. But that judgment is too crude to be a basis for medical decisions. Even the judgment that life is most valuable will not do; it makes a difference why one thinks life is of value. Imagine four physicians debating about the proper treatment for the patient in question. The first says, "Where there is life, there is hope. We all know of cases that have astounded us by wholly unexpected turns of improvement. We may not abandon this patient. For the good of this patient, we must continue to sustain his life as long as we can."

A second replies, "This patient is doomed. We all know that, unless we're kidding ourselves. Sometimes there are astounding improvements, but sometimes we know enough to know that a patient is on a one-way road. But we don't know very much about that new drug he's on, and the longer we keep him going, the more we stand to learn. And the residents and interns have an interest here, too. We owe it to them to let them see this thing play out all the way, see just what the limits are of what we can do here. So for the sake of medical research and medical education, we may not abandon this patient."

And the third: "Life is sacred. It is of value by itself, always and everywhere. It is not our role to decide when to end it. Our obligation is to prolong it as much as we can, without regard to the level or quality of the life. For the sake of ourselves as physicians and for the sake of life, we may not abandon this patient."

Finally, the fourth: "I agree that life is of great value. But I do not believe that it has that value intrinsically. Life has value because it is a prerequisite for everything else that is of value—it is a necessary condition for joy, pride in accomplishment, service to others, a sense of beauty, even self-indulgence or self-pity. It is the precondition of all experience, without which there is no intelligible sense in which value exists at all. But this patient is beyond experience or at least beyond any possible positive experience. He is in irreversible coma; he hasn't recognized anyone for days; he can no longer communicate; there is no source of satisfaction in his life, and there never again will be. So his life is not of any value to him, and it is inexcusable to preserve it because it is interesting or instructive to others. Life is the most precious thing there is because it is necessary for all experience. Where there can be no experience, there is no value to life. We are wasting a fortune and torturing his family. We have an obligation to stop prolonging the dying of this patient under the guise of saving lives.''

In this dispute, valuing life is something they all agree on, but because they value it in different ways and for different reasons, their behavioral decisions will differ. If the patient has been a lifelong advocate of the view that life is always and everywhere sacred above all, it would be better to let the third physician's decision prevail. But if the patient is the iconoclastic old philosopher at whose feet the fourth physician became persuaded of the strictly instrumental value of life, then it would be better to let the fourth physician prevail. This is simply to say that it is the patient's values that should dominate in such a case, yet in all likelihood they will not be well known, except, perhaps, as they can be taken as reflected in the views of the patient's wife. Further, to the extent that the physicians are unclear about what their own values are, why they hold them, and how they compare with the values that others hold, there is likely to be a randomness in the way decisions are made that depends on those values, and the patients of each physician will be treated in a slightly different way—in some cases perhaps in a wholly different way—because of differences in the values of the various physicians, not differences in the needs or values of the patients. A similar randomness will occur when the patient's values are unclear or unknown. So the more we as patients know about our own values, and the more physicians know about theirs, the better able we will be to devise structures of care that will adhere maximally to the values of the patients without unduly violating the values of the physicians, nurses, and others who provide that care.

PART TWO

Moral Decisions

5
Moral Conflict
and Moral Choice

I ONCE TAUGHT a course on moral issues in medicine that had, in the same class, both undergraduate philosophy students and students from the medical school. One day a physician from the university hospital presented to the class a description of a case that was confronting him at the moment—a case that seemed to present only morally troubling choices. The first student called upon to discuss the case launched a sustained inquiry into facts beyond those in the physician's initial presentation. "What is the family's economic status? Did you do a bone-marrow analysis?" And so on. The second student took a different approach. "We want to do the right thing here," he said. "And what that is depends on whether or not the consequences of our choice are the only morally relevant considerations." The first student had scorn for the second student's flight into abstraction. "This is a real case," he admonished. "A decision has to be made. We don't have time for another two thousand years of philosophical speculation, to see if you can resolve what you are still fighting about after the first two thousand years." And the second student had disdain for the first student's flight into empirical inquiry. "You seem to think," he derided, "that if you just do more tests and surveys and examinations, somehow you'll suddenly discover the right thing to do. But we already know what the issues are in this case; we know enough facts. What we have to decide is what is right, and you're not willing to face that question."

Both students were right in their criticisms; neither recognized the similarity in their avoidance behavior. Faced with the discomfort of a searingly tragic medical situation, the philosophy student fled to the comfortable refuge of philosophical abstractions. In a parallel way, the medical student plodded along the path of factual inquiry, shielding himself from the challenges of moral inquiry. And the physician pointed out that he had just a few minutes left with the class since he had to return to the hospital to deal with the case.

What the students gradually came to realize—sometimes grudgingly— is that issues of this sort cannot be successfully addressed within the confines of philosophy or within those of medicine. Instead, they require a steady interplay of both practical and theoretical considerations. Only after the two sets of students began each to develop some sense of the other's viewpoint did we begin to make a bit of progress. And so it is with our inquiries here.

Questions about what one ought to do are often questions of a practical sort. For example, whether to use a particular antibiotic, rather than some other one, will be decided on the basis of evidence about the comparative effectiveness of the two drugs for the infection, the patient's tolerance for the drugs, and possibly even questions of supply or cost. Such questions can be exceedingly complex and can sometimes involve conflicts of value that compound their complexity. Sometimes, however, they are straightforward; once one has the relevant facts, it is clear what ought to be done. It is clear, for example, that physicians who intend to reuse syringes should sterilize them between uses. But questions about what ought to be done are not always questions about the most effective path to a desired outcome; instead, they can be questions about what, from a moral point of view, is the right thing to do. Since much of what is philosophically most interesting about medical practice concerns uncertainty about what the morally right thing is to do, I want in this chapter to discuss various aspects of what moral judgments and moral dilemmas are like. After that it should be easier to understand what some of them are like in specifically medical contexts.

For many people, the hard question about morality is how to determine the right thing to do—its being taken for granted that doing the right thing is important. This was the view of Plato, who believed that doing a morally wrong thing was always an error of the understanding, the result of a failure to recognize the right course of action. It was impossible, he thought, to realize that an action was morally right and then to do otherwise.[1] His pupil Aristotle disagreed, thinking it common for people to know what was right and yet to do otherwise. For Aristotle, wrong action could result from weakness of the will—of motivation—even when one knew what one ought to do.[2] The question of the relationship between knowing what is right and wanting to do what is right has occupied philosophers through the ages but will not concern us here. Rather, I take it for granted that we share a concern with acting rightly and that we should therefore proceed directly to an inquiry into what acting rightly requires in the context of clinical medicine. To proceed otherwise would take us far afield because it is difficult at best, and perhaps impossible, to justify a commitment to morality to someone who does not share it. The person who asks, "Why should I be moral?" is asking a very difficult question—one I will not attempt to answer here.[3]

If we assume, then, that one wants to do what is right, what exactly is such moral behavior? Aristotle, writing about ethics, cautioned that one should not attempt to find more precision in the inquiry than the subject matter will allow.[4] At the outset it is unknown just how much precision that is; I therefore will approach the subject matter of morality by stages, characterizing it initially with a fairly rough sketch and subsequently seeking a higher level of precision.

Questions of morality are sometimes identified with questions of law, economics, psychology, or other areas. The connections are real enough, but morality is not simply a matter of these considerations, nor of sociology, prevailing public policy, history, or religion. All these areas may have some bearing on questions of morality; I'm sure that at least most of them do. But they are not the same as morality. This can be shown easily.

Consider first whether the question of what is required by morality is the same as the question of what is required by law. In many cases what the law requires is not completely clear. One common example is a law prohibiting vehicles from the park. Is this intended to exclude the delivery boy on a bicycle? What of the man in a wheelchair? We can clarify the legislation by rewording it to prohibit *motor* vehicles from the park. But then we may find that the man has revised his wheelchair while the legislature was revising the law; he has put a motor on it; it is now a motor vehicle! Further revisions of the law are possible, but the process is cumbersome, slow, costly, and unlikely to succeed. For events in the world unfold in ways that it is impossible ever fully to anticipate, and new situations arise which are neither clearly within nor clearly outside the scope of any given law.

It is far better to recognize the need for interpretation of law, for a process that can take into account such factors as legislative intent, the public interest, precedent, and common sense, as well as the text of the law in question, in determining what does and what does not fall within the scope of that law. Such a process is not morally neutral; turning to the law to solve questions of what to do can require that we confront morally significant questions in trying to understand the law—to which we turned in the hope of finding what is right to do.

Some of the time, however, the law is completely clear. A law absolutely prohibiting abortion under any circumstances would be such a law, unlike a law prohibiting abortion except when the life of the mother is seriously threatened. Even where the law specifies clearly what is required, however, the question of what is right to do remains, and we are compelled to ask whether the law should be broken or challenged by civil disobedience. Take a law strictly forbidding abortion as a case in point. In a state which had enacted such a law, a physician could be asked to abort the pregnancy of a thirteen-year-old victim of rape by an escapee from a state institution for those among the criminally insane who have serious heritable diseases. In such a case the physician would face a moral question—whether to aid the patient despite the law or to obey the law despite the very strong case for aborting the pregnancy.

Notice that I have not said what the physician should do; I have said only that the physician faces a moral question. There is a decision to be made, which different physicians might well make differently. I claim only that it is a significant question to ask what the physician ought to do in such a situation. Yet it is *not* a significant question to ask what the law requires in such a situation; that is a trivial question because the law is completely explicit on the issue. Since one of these two questions is significant, and the other is not, these must be two *different* questions. Thus, to ask what is morally required is to ask a different question from the question of what is legally required. This shows that morality is not simply a question of what the law specifies but is something other than law.

This is not to say that the law is morally irrelevant. On the contrary, the legal facts typically have substantial bearing on our moral deliberations, and should. My point is only that those moral deliberations are sometimes not settled entirely by reference to the law—which shows that whatever morality is, it must be something that is not identical to conformity to law.

A similar argument shows that morality and economics are not identical. Economics often considers questions closely related to moral issues, and it can be tempting to approach a morally troubling situation in economic terms. Production, supply, demand, price, and distribution all are related to questions of social justice, equality, and the satisfaction of human needs and wants. Nonetheless, the economic aspects of a case alone do not entail any moral conclusion about what, all things considered, is right to do. The question of the withdrawal of life-extending treatment—of "pulling the plug," to use that deplorable colloquialism—is easily resolved on economic grounds in the typical case. It is almost always cheaper, more economically efficient, to "pull the plug" when a patient's prospects for significant recovery are slight. Yet we cannot help wondering whether doing so is right. And no matter what the answer, the very meaningfulness of the question shows that rightness is something other than economic efficiency alone. So moral judgments are not merely economic judgments.

Similarly, what is psychologically most comfortable or most ennobling, what is sociologically most common, what accords with prevailing public policy, what is in keeping with historical precedent or tradition, and what conforms to the strictures of whatever religious viewpoint, if any, one favors can all be questioned on moral grounds. So the moral dimensions of a situation are not simply the same as the dimensions that fall within the scope of these other areas.

Morality as a domain of judgment is different from any other. To say this, however, is not to explain what does fall within that domain or to deny that morality is closely linked with other areas. The question of what the relationship is between the morality of a situation, on the one hand, and the facts of the situation—that is, the economic, legal, psychological, religious, and other facts—on the other, has been the subject of enduring debate within philosophy. Some writers have held that moral judgments stand entirely apart from judgments of any other sort. But a larger number of writers have believed that moral judgments do depend in some way on the facts of the matter—that while morality may not be *simply* a question of law, economics, psychology, or any other single discipline, the legal, economic, psychological, and other such facts nonetheless together influence what the appropriate moral judgment is in any situation. I shall return to the question of what sorts of facts are morally relevant and how they relate to moral judgment. But it is time first to say something more positive about the subject matter of moral philosophy.

Moral judgments involve an elusive, complex, yet centrally important cluster of concepts: justice, human dignity, rights, the resolution of conflicts among rights, equity, integrity, virtue, duty, and the rightness or wrongness of action. It is not easy to clarify what is meant by all that language, and I will not attempt to do so here. I merely want it clear that these are the sorts of issues involved in the making of moral judgments. As our discussion proceeds, we will have occasion to consider some of these concepts and how they relate to decisions in medical practice. And it would surely be an advantage to have, at the outset, a clear understanding of all of them—or even of some of them. But it is unfortunately impossible to gain that advantage. It is worth considering why not.

If you and I do not share a common understanding of the language I write, then I will fail at communicating effectively to you. You may wonder, therefore, why I do not simply define those terms that will play a crucial role in our discussions—terms like *right* and *wrong*, *just* and *unjust*. Then, when I use such morally significant language, there would be no confusion about what is meant. This approach is often suggested by students. Under heavy pressure themselves to be clear and precise in their use of language, they naturally want the instructor to be clear as well and, in particular, to define the centrally important terms. The suggestion is understandable but futile. The definition of moral terms is not, and cannot be, simply a result of clarification of language—of linguistic investigation. Rather, the definition of moral terms has substantive moral content. Let me illustrate.

Suppose I claim that the word *right* means the same as the expression *conforms to the wishes of the majority*. I have then put forward a moral theory about what right action is. Another person may object to that moral theory, claiming that what is right is what conforms to the will of a god in which he believes, but I do not. He, then, holds that *right* means "conforms to the teachings of Divinus." Is our quarrel one about words or substance? Do we share an understanding of the word *right* yet disagree about how to apply it, or do we have no common understanding of the word?

Compare this situation with one in which I believe that tetracycline is more effective against a particular strain of bacterium than is penicillin, but you believe that penicillin is the more effective. You and I might agree completely on what the word *effective* means, although we disagree about the drug to which it is more properly applied. We could then conduct experiments that would eliminate our dispute, confirming which of the drugs better satisfies our mutually accepted understanding of what effectiveness in drug therapy is. Our dispute is not about theories of pharmaceutical effectiveness; it is just a disagreement about a particular application of a term we both understand.

The dispute about what counts as right action is not of this sort. It is a dispute about the very substance of morality, reflected in our *advocacy* of different definitions for the term *right*. To adopt a definition for the term *right*, used in its moral sense, is thus to reach a morally significant conclusion. That is why no such definition can simply be stipulated at the outset of our inquiry.

It would be a grievous error to overreact to this point, concluding that we do not understand moral language. This is a common reaction in introductory ethics classes to the discovery that an acceptable definition of moral terms is beyond reach. It goes like this: I ask the students to give some examples of actions they consider right and others they consider wrong. They readily comply; it is an easy task. I then ask them to explain what they mean by calling certain actions right, and chaos emerges. Some express the view that right actions are the ones that people ought to do, thereby sweeping the problem of clarifying rightness under the equally unclear carpet of obligation. Others offer religious views, or speak of the greatest good of the greatest number, or take refuge in the position that doing what seems best at the time is always right, or give up entirely their position of a few moments earlier that there is any understandable distinction between right and wrong. If I ask them at that point to set aside the problem of explaining the difference between rightness and wrongness and invite them simply to tell me what the word *right* means when, as speakers of English, they use it to describe certain actions and not others, they see that trying to answer the question of definition involves them in defending a theory of morality. Recognizing that they simply cannot define the moral language they have been using, they are typically all too ready to agree that they do not understand that language at all.

The mistake lies in the assumption that we have no understanding of what we cannot define. To dispel the confusion, we consider three examples. First, we consider a definition of *sibling*. Most of the students understand this word and can correctly define it as synonymous with *brother or sister*. So we have an example of a word we do understand, along with its definition. Next, I offer a definition for them to consider: A trochilidist is one who studies hummingbirds. I ask them to tell me whether that definition is correct or not; they are unable to do so because entirely lacking any understanding of the word *trochilidae*, they simply have no basis for accepting or rejecting the definition I have provided. They recognize that only if they had some such understanding could they have any opinion about whether my definition was linguistic information or fraud.

Finally, I offer them a definition of *right* as applied to the moral character of actions. An action is right, I explain, if it is performed east of the Mississippi, wrong otherwise. They immediately reject my definition as incorrect. I then try another: *Right* means "benefits the members of the party in power." This, too, they reject, realizing that an action can benefit the party in power and still be wrong. At this point most of them realize that they can properly reject these fraudulent definitions only because they already have a partial understanding of the correct use of moral language. They may not understand it well enough to define it as they can define *sibling*, but they understand it considerably better than they understand *trochilidist*, which is simply not a part of their functional vocabulary. And that partial understanding, limited and erratic though it may be, constitutes an important foundation for the pursuit of moral inquiry.

One basis for rejecting a proposed definition of a moral term, then, is that the definition is in conflict with our rough understanding of how moral language is properly used. That is how we know that whatever rightness is, it cannot be simply whatever benefits the party in power. This kind of argument rests on an appeal to our moral intuitions—our deeply held convictions and deeply felt attitudes about rightness and wrongness. Yet although people feel strongly, they often feel differently about what is right. How, then, can moral intuitions be a court of appeal without the result being confusion? In the case of abortion, for example, people on various sides of the debate (there are, after all, more than two) have intensely strong intuitions about what is right and what is wrong. Under such circumstances how can moral intuitions possibly be of value in the effort to decide what is right?

One reason why moral philosophy is so hard is that a case or situation tends to be the focus of sustained attention only if it is difficult and contested. If it is clear to everyone that an action is wrong, there is no debate about it, and it will not likely engage the interest of philosophers or of anyone else. But if a case divides opinion and creates painful conflict within individuals, then it becomes a typical object of philosophical inquiry. No wonder there is frustration in doing moral philosophy, when it is mainly the frustrating cases that get the attention! But there are clear and simple cases, too, and their importance is easily overlooked. We are not in moral conflict, for example, about the rightness of mugging octogenarian pensioners for sport, of boiling babies for bouillon, or of punting puppies for exercise. That these actions are wrong is clear and undisputed, and the judgments to that effect constitute a part of the hard data of moral philosophy. Not all our moral intuitions are about hard cases. The cases that are easy, undisputed, unrelated to any real sense of conflict, are the fixed points in our evidence about moral judgment.

Any theory about the difference between right and wrong must pass the test of agreement with these fixed points. Indeed, we have more confidence in these particular judgments than we do in any general theory that conflicts with them. If a theory accords well with our intuitions at this level, we can then consider the result of applying it to cases in which we have less clarity and less confidence in our intuitive judgments. The hope that motivates much inquiry in moral philosophy is that if a theory of the difference between right and wrong corresponds well to our judgments where they are clear, it will help us decide—it will help us form judgments—in those cases which are contested. So we recognize that moral intuitions can help us achieve greater clarity about difficult cases, but only as part of a complex array of considerations that must all be assessed together. With this methodological point in mind, let us turn at last to the question of what sorts of actions are right.

Two major traditions in moral philosophy—different viewpoints in thinking about ethical questions—divide over the issue of whether and to what extent the actual or expected consequences of an action determine its moral quality. One tradition includes those who hold that the moral character of an act depends on its consequences in whole or in part. We call such a position consequentialist. This tradition is exemplified by the utilitarian view of right action, most notably associated with Jeremy Bentham, John Stuart Mill, and a long line of Mill's intellectual descendants.[5] Utilitarianism holds that actions are right if—and only if—they produce the greatest happiness (or utility) for the greatest number of persons. Other views than utilitarianism can be consequentialist, too, however. For example, the erroneous view that those actions are right which maximize beauty in the world, quite apart from the amount of suffering they cause and the amount of happiness or benefit associated with that beauty, would be a consequentialist, but nonutilitarian, theory.

The other major tradition in moral philosophy comprises ethical theories which hold that the moral status of an action is independent of its consequences. This sort of moral theory is exemplified by the views of Immanuel Kant and those who write in his tradition.[6] For Kant, actions are right or wrong independently of the consequences; to be right, an action must have been done from a certain sort of motive. Moral theories that categorize certain classes of action as simply being right or wrong, such as is done by any list of commandments or prescriptions, are also typically nonconsequentialist. Thus, some traditional orthodoxies admonish us to refrain utterly from acts of certain kinds, such as killing, stealing, or lying, on the ground that they are wrong simply by virtue of the kinds of acts that they are. These nonconsequentialist theories are called formalist or deontological theories.

The apparent simplicity of utilitarianism as a moral theory is deceptive. On the surface the theory seems clear and compelling. What could be morally superior to that act which produces more good for more people than any other? But various problems with the theory quickly emerge. First, there are problems internal to the theory—that is, problems in making sense of what it really says. On the one hand, it requires us to maximize the production of happiness; on the other hand, it seems to take distribution into account in speaking of the greatest number. But these two considerations can pull in opposite directions. It may be that in some circumstances we can maximize happiness only by reducing the number of people who are benefited. It is not at all clear how utilitarianism requires us to handle such a situation.

A second internal problem is that of identifying consequences. If the moral character of an action depends on its consequences, it becomes important to know what consequences will flow, or have flown, from each action. But predicting the future is notoriously hard. It is even difficult to tell what is true of the past. If I carelessly give you the wrong medicine and in dealing with the resulting illness, a bright young doctor makes an important discovery that saves many lives, is that discovery one of the consequences of my action? Causal chains are frustratingly resistant to clarification, and it is never easy to be sure what we are talking about when we speak of the consequences of an action. Yet utilitarianism requires us to base our assessment of actions on just such talk.

A third internal problem is that the theory requires us to make comparative judgments about human happiness. Yet it is not obvious that such comparisons can be made in any adequate way. You may exhibit more overt glee than your neighbor, but is it not possible that behind his veneer of restraint he knows a joy that far transcends what prompts your more visible delight? How are we to tell which actions produce the most happiness when it seems impossible to compare one person's happiness with another's?

Despite these problems, utilitarianism has had many defenders, and much of the literature revolves around attempts to fashion a form of utilitarianism that surmounts these difficulties. The more serious challenge to utilitarianism comes from a different direction, however.

The external problems are those that remain once one assumes it possible to understand just what utilitarianism requires and further assumes that it is possible to act in accordance with those requirements. Even then, the charge goes, utilitarianism will not do because it is itself morally unacceptable. Utilitarianism is a theory that defines *right action* as *maximizing* action; it places no constraints on the means to that maximization. It is possible to imagine situations in which the greatest good for the greatest number could be achieved by punishing an innocent man, enslaving a powerless minority, or committing an undetected crime.

These actions are wrong despite their consequences, yet the utilitarian is bound to praise them. Thus, utilitarianism is refuted, according to this line of attack.

The utilitarians have fought back with the claim that such criticism misses the mark because it is based on a misunderstanding of the theory it attacks. That misunderstanding, it is claimed, results from taking the principle of utilitarianism to be a principle for evaluating actions when, in fact, it is a principle for evaluating moral guidelines or rules. A moral rule will be accepted, according to this defense of utilitarianism, if its adoption is conducive to producing the greatest happiness for the greatest number. Thus, for utilitarian reasons, we have rules against framing the innocent, enslaving our fellowmen, and committing crimes. So the utilitarian need not endorse such actions after all.

The version of utilitarianism according to which it is individual actions that are to be judged by the utilitarian principle is called, unsurprisingly, *act* utilitarianism. The version according to which actions are judged by rules which are themselves measured against the utilitarian standard is called *rule* utilitarianism. Recent disputes in moral philosophy have focused on the question of whether act utilitarianism and rule utilitarianism are genuinely different—whether one version can escape objections that are telling against the other—and that question remains unresolved. Critics of utilitarianism continue to attack it; its sympathizers continue to devise reformulations of the theory that they hope will be immune to the attacks. But although utilitarianism receives much attention within moral philosophy, it is not the only focus of attention. There are non-consequentialist theories as well, contending for prominence.

Plato believed that actions were right if they corresponded to the Good, an ideal that existed independently of any human actions or material objects. The Platonic theory of right action was so obscure and unrelated to actual moral concerns that it was soundly criticized by Aristotle as being irrelevant to human moral deliberation—and therefore deficient as moral philosophy. In Plato's view, rightness was not dependent on the consequences of action; the problem was making sense of what Plato thought it did depend on. (We will consider Aristotle's view of morality later, noting for now merely that he believed the essence of virtue to be rational control of desires, leading to moderation in action.)

Early systems of ethics based on theological beliefs also provide examples of deontological ethical theories. If an action breaks one of the Ten Commandments, there is no question of whether some useful purpose was thereby served; it is a violation, a wrongdoing, simply because a commandment has been broken. Even a theory that had a place within it for consideration of extenuating circumstances would be deontological if it were based on a set of commandments, provided only that the primary basis of moral judgment was conformity to the commandments.

For Kant, the test of an action's morality is the motive from which it springs. Good intentions are not enough, however. To be right, an action must have been done out of a sense of duty, a desire to do the right thing solely because it is right. Further, strict logical conditions limit the choice of actions. Each intentional action conforms to some principle. For example, if I break my promise to you because it is profitable to do so, the principle according to which I am acting allows selective promise breaking. But that cannot be my duty, according to Kant, because of a point of logic. Kant believed that such a principle leads to inconsistency. If I act on such a principle, I must acknowledge the right of anyone else to act on the same principle. But that would mean that people could break their promises whenever there was advantage to be gained by doing so. If that were the case, then there could be no institution of promising; the very possibility of making a promise depends on its being generally understood that one does have an obligation to keep one's promises. In effect, to act on a principle that allows selective promise breaking is to hold that one has no obligation to do what one has an obligation to do. Promise breaking is therefore wrong, always and everywhere, regardless of its consequences.

A second version of Kant's ethical theory—one he claims is equivalent to the first—rests on the principle that one must treat other people always as ends unto themselves and never as means only. If, to continue the example, I break my promise to you for my own profit, I am misusing you, violating your rights for my purposes. I am failing to respect you as an end; I am treating you merely as a means to the furtherance of my own goals. Such action, according to Kant, is always wrong, no matter what the consequences.

This is not to say I cannot justifiably treat others as means. For example, if I want my house painted, I can hire a house painter. He then functions as a means to the achievement of my goal. But he does so freely, acting in pursuit of goals of his own. So I have not treated him as a means only. Rather, I have enlisted his efforts by linking my aspirations with his, respecting his status as an autonomous agent who can freely accept or decline my offer. If I force him to paint the house, however, I have treated him as a means only; I have used him, much as I might use a brush or ladder, violating his dignity as a person.

Kantian morality is austere and unforgiving. It requires strict adherence to principles that draw sharp lines between right and wrong. Duty is clear and simple. Never lie; always keep your promises; never violate the dignity of another. There is no room for explanation of the special circumstance or for suspending a moral rule because of the consequences that will follow if it is not suspended in unusual circumstances.

Unusual circumstances, however, are the stuff of which moral dilemmas are made. I can unwittingly find myself in a situation in which the only way I can keep a promise is by telling a lie. No matter that I should have avoided such situations. What do I do? For the act utilitarian, the answer is easy. I do the thing that maximizes happiness. But Kant gives us no answer at all. He fails to consider the resolution of moral conflict, writing as if the choices we face are like the choice between keeping a promise and breaking it for selfish reasons, rather than the choice between keeping a promise and remaining honest.

Despite such difficulties, Kant has been a moral theorist of towering influence. His resounding defense of the inviolable dignity of each person is a landmark in moral argument; his principle that one must never treat another as a means only, but always as an end unto himself, captures a profound moral insight that lies at the heart of the most powerful objections to consequentialist morality.

Much of the history of moral philosophy deals with the tension between these two basic points of view about the moral importance of consequences and with the attempts on the part of moral theorists to resolve the dispute or strike some sort of plausible balance. Clearly we do have strong temptation to hold the consequences of actions to be relevant to their moral status, and thus, consequentialist moral theories have substantial and sustained appeal. However, they have not become fully dominant precisely because we also believe that there is something morally lacking in an approach that focuses solely on consequences and refuses to acknowledge that certain kinds of actions are simply wrong.

Both consequentialists and nonconsequentialists typically share the view that each person is of equal value as regards that elusive cluster of issues that constitute the subject matter of moral philosophy—right action, moral worth, human rights, justice. Thus, for Mill and the utilitarians, it is the productivity of happiness and the avoidance of pain that count; but everyone's happiness is equally important, and everyone's pain is equally lamentable. And for Kant, moral action must be guided by a principle that one can logically will to be followed by all other persons, without exception. Indeed, it is widely taken to be a criterion of adequacy for any moral theory that it apply equally to all similarly situated persons. Thus, if telling a lie is wrong regardless of the circumstances, it is wrong not merely for you but for me and for anyone else. And if there are some circumstances under which, on utilitarian grounds or any others, it is morally permissible to tell a lie, then it is as permissible for you under those circumstances as it is for me or for anyone else. We thus find endorsement in moral philosophy of the requirement that to be taken seriously as a moral principle, a principle must be applicable equally to all persons as moral agents. That is, what one may do (or is prohibited from doing) all may do (or are prohibited from doing) under circumstances that are similar in morally relevant respects.

This requirement serves to test the moral acceptability of principles concerning how people may, must, or are forbidden to act, and it is essentially a requirement based on a widely shared conviction to the effect that morality allows no bias toward or prejudice against anyone to the advantage or disadvantage of anyone else. Not all theories satisfy this requirement, so it is a requirement that has real force. It rules out, for example, the old notion of perfectionism—the view that what is right is what serves the interests of the finest exemplars of the human species. According to that view, if you have to grind a thousand peasants into the dust to enrich the life of one talented aristocrat, you should grind away. The right course of action is not that which treats people equally or well or maximizes happiness; it is that course of action which produces the occasional Bach, Newton, or Picasso—and this because the ultimate good has to do with perfecting the species or upholding some high standard of achievement. Such a position, advocated by Nietzsche, also had proponents among the ancient Greeks and the nineteenth-century English aristocracy.

Such theories go against the grain because of their apparent injustice. But clarification of the concept of justice is no less a task than that of clarifying the concept of right action. Indeed, Plato's *Republic*, probably the most famous and important single work in the history of philosophy, takes the concept of justice as its primary focus. The inquiry proceeds by the attempt to discover what the correct definition of the term *just* is. Each definition that is considered is a different theory of justice; an acceptable definition is sought as the culmination of the inquiry, not as a prerequisite to beginning it.

We, too, will be concerned with justice, especially in the delivery of health care. So it behooves us to spend some time considering some competing theories of what justice is. There is no shortage of them. For our purposes, it will suffice to consider three of them in historical order. The first is that held by Mill, for whom justice was a subsidiary moral concept. That is, for Mill, the principles of justice are those guidelines to behavior that we have learned, over the ages, are most important in leading people to act in a utilitarian way.[7] For example, it is unjust to punish an innocent man for a crime we know he did not commit, even if there is some social benefit to be gained by convicting him, and this is a reflection of the fact that respecting the rule that requires us to punish only the guilty will lead to maximizing happiness in the long run. Justice, for Mill, is a value that is derivative from the utilitarian principle and hence can never be in conflict with it. The right thing to do will always be just and will always be that which maximizes happiness.

Mill's view has been challenged by the observation that there can arise situations in which the action that maximizes happiness is plainly unjust. Consider this example. A surgeon has five patients, each of whom faces death because of the failure of a different organ. In each case a transplant would save the patient, but there are no donor organs available. Suddenly the surgeon is called to deal with an emergency—a sixth patient who has been in a serious accident. The surgeon discovers that he can easily save the new patient, whose prospects for complete recovery are excellent, although everyone else erroneously thinks the case is hopeless. But the surgeon realizes that if he deliberately fails at the attempt, he can then take the five needed organs from the new patient—who, being unconscious, will never know the difference—and save the lives of all five of the other patients. If we assume that the surgeon can circumvent legal jeopardy, the utilitarian principle plainly seems to require that he perform such action. Yet his doing so seems equally plainly to be an unjust violation of the rights of the new patient. The defender of utilitarianism is faced with two choices: He can argue that his example misrepresents the utilitarian position, or he can accept the example, claiming that the surgeon should indeed take such action, which we only perceive as unjust because of a benighted refusal to embrace utilitarianism as the true moral view. Neither line of defense has been entirely successful—though both have their advocates—and utilitarianism as a theory of justice has failed to win universal endorsement.

Despite the criticisms of utilitarianism, it has been the dominant moral theory for most of the last century largely because even its most effective critics have failed to offer an equally appealing theory to displace it. Very recent work in political philosophy has altered the situation, however. Two contemporary discussions of justice have received widespread attention and have rekindled intense interest in moral and political philosophy not only within professional philosophical circles but within a much broader readership.

The first of these discussions appears in *A Theory of Justice*, by John Rawls.[8] No other work of philosophy in modern times has received as much attention so soon after its publication; now, a decade later, there are many dissertations, articles, reviews, books, and anthologies based on the Rawlsian corpus. We will not consider the theory in detail, nor discuss the elaborate argument that Rawls offers in defense of it. The conclusions alone are of considerable interest; it will suffice to review them.

Rawls's theory of justice yields two basic principles. The first is the Principle of Liberty, which requires the just society to provide each individual with the maximum amount of personal freedom that is compatible with a system of like liberty for all.[9] It is a simple principle, really, which reflects both the desire to accord each individual the best possible approximation to maximum liberty and the realization that to give any individual total liberty is on that account to limit the liberty of others. So each person's liberty must be limited to some extent to protect the liberty of others, and the most just arrangement is that in which the limits on liberty are imposed equally on everyone. This first principle does not pertain to the distribution of goods or services; it simply states that each person is free to do as he or she pleases so long as that does not constrain the liberty of others. The point of the principle is freedom and the protection of individual rights of action.

The second principle is the Difference Principle, which requires that opportunities, goods, and all the benefits of social organization, both tangible and intangible, be distributed equally—except that it is justifiable to deviate from equality when the benefits of the resulting unequal distribution accrue maximally to the least advantaged.[10] We can illustrate the force of this second principle with a simple example. Imagine an isolated community, seeking after a shipwreck to establish a social order on an island that is otherwise uninhabited. One horse survives along with the passengers. Who is to get the horse? An advocate of equality argues that each of them is equally entitled to the horse and suggests that they take turns so that each of them has the same amount of time to use it. The Rawlsian then objects, pointing out a better solution that is also just. One of the survivors is a physician, he notes, whose services are of particular importance to all those in the community. If the physician is given the horse, that is a special advantage and a deviation from equality. But the deviation is to everyone's advantage; it results in their all having access to medical care. In particular, and this is essential, it is especially to the benefit of the least advantaged members of the society—those who are least well and who perhaps have little to contribute to the community. So this is a preferable distribution, to which everyone could rationally agree in his own interest, even though it deviates from equality. (The idea of selecting principles that every rational, self-interested person would be willing to accept is crucial to Rawls's method of arguing for his theory.) Inequality is therefore not necessarily inequity, according to Rawls, but is justifiable when it benefits the least advantaged.

This is, of course, just a glimpse of Rawls's work. Still, even this glimpse will be useful as we compare his theory with others. For example, it might be thought that Rawls is a utilitarian, defending the unequal distribution because it is in the best interests of the community as a whole. But that interpretation is explicitly rejected by Rawls. For what is in the best interests of the community as a whole may increase the deprivation of the least advantaged and would therefore be unjustified for Rawls even as it is applauded by the utilitarian. Rather, Rawls accepts deviations from equality only on the ground that they benefit the least advantaged, not on the ground that they increase the average or total level of well-being.

A second contemporary theory provides a powerful criticism of both the utilitarian point of view and the Rawlsian theory. In *Anarchy, State and Utopia*,[11] Robert Nozick holds that subject to a few important constraints, one is entitled to whatever one has. What you come by honestly is yours to do with as you will, and the plight of others is not relevant. What is coming by something honestly? If I steal what is yours or get it by fraud or deceit, it does not become mine. It is mine, however, if I buy it from someone whose it was to sell or if it is given to me as a gift by one whose it was to give. And it is mine if I acquire it initially, as when I go onto unowned land and construct something of natural materials found there. I have made it, mixed my labor with materials that were unowned, and it therefore becomes my own.[12] Redistribution of wealth or goods by government action is an unjustified violation of individual rights, although people are free to contribute voluntarily to redistributional organizations.

Utopia is, then, a minimal state, close to anarchy. It is not quite anarchy because there is a proper role for government's ensuring that acquisitions and transfers are legitimate and that people do not have their goods taken unjustifiably. Unsophisticated defenders of laissez-faire free-enterprise capitalism love Nozick's view. But they do not read him carefully enough. For there is in his theory the notion of corrective redistribution, which may require drastic government action. If one considers the history of how people presently owning things came to acquire them, it becomes clear that there are few legitimate holdings. The wealth of America is based largely on stolen land, slave labor, and deception, and hence there are in Nozick's work the seeds of a radical view of governmentally imposed redistribution. But he does not spell this out; indeed, one reason the book is so unsatisfying is that he does not spell out anything in significant detail.

Nonetheless, the theory contains arguments that give one pause about the Rawlsian point of view, and more. Most theories of justice describe certain states of affairs as being just or unjust depending on the pattern of distribution of goods and services. Thus, to advocate a distribution to each equally is to advocate the pattern that egalitarians say is the only just distribution. To distribute to each according to his needs, or in the way that maximizes happiness, is to adopt other patterns. Nozick says that what is wrong with all these theories is not that they rely on the wrong pattern, but that they construe justice as a property of patterns of distribution at all.

Assume that you respect individual freedom. Assume also that people are entitled to what they have since the distribution accords strictly with your conception of justice. A dilemma emerges. Wilt Chamberlain is superb at making a spherical object go through a hoop ten feet above the ground. Lots of people get very excited about that fact and are willing to allocate a small bit of their wealth to see him do it. Should they be free to do so? Nozick argues that any restriction preventing them from making such an arrangement would be a massive intrusion into simple interpersonal transactions. But if enough people are willing to spend even a very small amount to see Chamberlain play, he can amass great wealth. Then a redistribution has resulted from the voluntary actions of people whose goods were justly held. Chamberlain has, say, a million dollars in his pocket, and a lot of people have just a tiny bit less in theirs. Is this new distribution just or unjust?

If you are wedded to the view that a just distribution requires everyone to have the same amount, the new distribution is clearly not just. Indeed, if you believe that justice requires any particular distribution, you must so structure society that these voluntary transactions cannot take place. That, says Nozick, is incompatible with our convictions about individual freedom. That is, we can maintain equality, or any other pattern of distribution, only in a state of tyranny.

Contrast the situation with one in which Chamberlain has a million dollars in his pocket because he is skilled at picking the pockets of other people. The resulting distribution is precisely what it was in the first situation, yet is obviously not just. What distinguishes the former situation from the latter is in the history—not in the resulting pattern of distribution, but in how that pattern came into being. If there is one primary message in Nozick's theory, it is that justice is a historical matter—a function not solely of how goods and services are distributed but of how that distribution came about. And there is not a trace in Rawls, or in most of the other writers on justice, of acknowledgment of that history. In short, Nozick is saying that every other theory of justice is itself unjust because it eliminates entirely the concept of desert, of having what you have because in some sense you deserve it.

I want to stand back from these theories of justice now and ask what we have when we are given such a theory. Rawls and Nozick provide different arguments with respect to rather large-scale objectives. Rawls seeks to provide a framework for the basic structure of social organization at a more fundamental level even than the design of a constitution. He explicitly says that his theory provides the constraints within which the constitution of a government can be written. Subsequent stages in the establishment of a social order involve writing a constitution, writing legislation in accordance with that constitution, and then adopting principles and procedures for enforcement and for adjudication of disputes. Those steps follow a long way down from the two basic principles of justice. Nozick, too, gives us a fundamental kind of viewpoint but says nothing substantial about the real world in which the transgression of principles requires rectification.

What do people ask of these theories? Often, that they provide solutions to very specific problems. I have heard this question, for example: "I am a hospital social worker. I have to choose between working with a poor Appalachian family and a poor Black family. These are their circumstances. . . . What does Rawls say about what I should do?" The answer is: Nothing. Rawls does not say anything about such specific choices. Rather, he is talking about very basic constraints on the shape of social organization, not about daily transactions. He does not say anything about what to do with a severely handicapped neonate or about how physicians should allocate their time or about any other comparably specific problem. Nor does Nozick, who also offers a theory from which very little follows about most specific problems that one confronts. Can we nonetheless somehow gain illumination of specific problems from considering these theories?

Doing so requires interpreting these theories of justice as points of view with respect to smaller-scale problems, not as axioms from which theorems can be derived. By taking a theory in this way, one can at least use it heuristically. Consider this example. In the debate about whether or not the United States should build a supersonic transport, some people pointed out that an infinitesimal percentage of the population would ever fly on such a craft. "The SST won't be good for the country to invest in," they claimed, "because so few people will use it." The response of the proponents of the SST was that the objection reflected a misunderstanding: "That's not why it's valuable—because it will enable the rich to go to Paris for lunch and be back in time for dinner. The point is that it will take jobs to build the SST, employment for lots of plain folks like the guy who sweeps the aircraft plant. And there will be benefits to everyone from better accessibility for government and corporate leaders. Progress of all sorts—political, industrial, scientific, and cultural—will be enhanced. The world is better off if world leaders can meet face-to-face on a few hours' notice." This answer is straightforwardly utilitarian; although the SST itself would transport only a few, the general welfare is maximized by our developing it.

But what does it do for the migratory farm worker? The utilitarian defender of the SST can say without embarrassment that it doesn't do much for the migratory farm worker because the case is strong enough if it maximizes the general welfare by doing good for a large number of other people. There is a Rawlsian rejoinder to the utilitarian, however: "Perhaps there is a utilitarian defense of the SST, but utilitarian arguments are erroneous. The fact that something maximizes social utility is itself not adequate justification for doing it. Slavery might under some circumstances maximize total happiness. For example, certain jobs are hard to get done in an affluent, educated society; as educational opportunity increases, they may get harder still. If we have good schooling for everyone, there may be no one left to collect the garbage. We could then take five percent of the population and enslave them to do the menial tasks, being careful to use modern techniques of behavior conditioning to ensure that they remain happy. We'll condition them not to have aspirations that transcend their lowly lot in life, so they won't suffer.

"This may be the utilitarian thing to do," the Rawlsian continues, "but we reject the plan because it violates individual rights. Utilitarian arguments do not always carry the day. So don't ask simply what the SST can do for business or even for the population on the whole. Ask what it will do for the least advantaged. Look at the people worst off in our society, and ask what an investment in the SST will do for them. And if the answer is that it will not help them, then the fact that it benefits the upper and middle classes is an argument against it because it moves them all up, increasing inequality by leaving the people at the bottom even further behind the social mainstream. It is therefore wrong, and we should invest resources, instead, in something that would accrue to the benefit of the least advantaged. Always the most important criterion is bringing the bottom up."

Here the Rawlsian is reflecting Rawls's conviction that we should judge the justice of a society by the way it treats those whom it treats least well—not by the standard of living of the typical member, not by the aggregate well-being, not the average or the GNP, but by how people do at the bottom. The Rawlsian approach on the SST is therefore very different from that of the utilitarian; it directs our attention to a different cluster of issues. Indeed, each of the theories we have sketched emphasizes different factors as being crucial in the assessment of the justice of a situation, and each thus sets for us a different agenda of inquiry. For the utilitarian, the amount of happiness produced is first among the morally relevant factors in judging the justice of a distribution or the rightness of an action. For Nozick, it is the protection of individual rights and the history of transfers of goods. And for Rawls it is respect for liberty and the interests of the least advantaged. Bearing these theories in mind will not by itself lead to the solution of specific moral dilemmas, but it will help us identify what prominent moral philosophers have thought are the most important factors in making moral judgments.

It is important to clarify a possible confusion here. We began by asking about the difference between doing the right thing and doing something wrong, and then the discussion turned to a consideration of questions of justice. For Mill and the utilitarians, justice was a matter of morality, and the question of what was right was more basic than the question of what was just. Not so for Rawls; he holds that justice is the first virtue of social institutions but does not by any means exhaust the whole of morality. In particular, considerations of justice will not, for Rawls, by themselves determine what constitutes right action. Similarly, Nozick offers a discussion of justice that does not pretend to be a theory of moral action but is an account with more limited scope. Further, there are theories of right action, such as that of Immanuel Kant, which say little about justice or social organization.

This abundance of theories about matters of moral judgment may give the newcomer to moral philosophy an impression of chaos, of an array of viewpoints so diverse and numerous as to lead one to despair of gaining from their study any clarification of the moral problems that one has to face amidst the affairs of practical life. That each of these theories is the result of sustained and serious inquiry does not help the situation. Yet despair is premature; in fact, there is a sort of order and reason that emerges from the apparent confusion, as we will see in chapters 7 and 8, on Resolving Moral Conflict.

It is worth noting that moral philosophy arises in the first place out of moral dilemma. Aristotle rightly observed that philosophy begins in wonder;[13] moral philosophy begins in wondering about what is right to do. Such puzzlements arise in two different ways. Sometimes we disagree with the judgments that other people make about what is right to do, and a conflict about moral judgment appears. And sometimes we are in conflict ourselves, seeing a contemplated action as right in some ways and wrong in others, so that whatever we decide causes us to be uncomfortable about the decision we have made. Either sort of conflict, considered reflectively, can generate the first rumblings of moral philosophy. Since moral philosophy arises out of conflict and reflects our ambivalence about what to do in what are typically very troubling situations, it should be no surprise that the principles and theories that emerge retain the sense of tension that prompts the inquiry in the first place. What is perhaps surprising is that we can learn something from it all that can help us understand what we ought to do.

Finally, before we return to specifically medical issues, I want to offer a few words about methodology. I have used examples here and there that will seem rather farfetched to many a reader. No surgeon, some will say, would ever consider plundering one patient to gain organs for the benefit of others; it is a situation that does not arise and hence is not a real problem. No shipwrecked group ever deliberates about the principles of justice that should determine who gets the horse, another may complain. These are false concerns. Such examples are artificial, to be sure. But they are designed to isolate in a clear way the relevant features of some particular theory, and their artificiality is an unavoidable consequence of the simplicity that results from filtering out the complexities of real life.

Nothing in this approach is peculiar to philosophy; indeed, it is quite standard even in a "hard science" like physics. The frictionless plane and the perfectly inelastic sphere that are so familiar in the teaching of elementary mechanics do not exist. No matter; when one wants to focus on clarification of the basic principles, friction need not be taken into account. It is what would happen in the absence of friction that must be first understood; later the complexities of the real world, in which friction is ever-present, can be added to the deliberation. Our situation is quite the same, and there is no good reason to hold philosophy to a higher standard of correspondence with reality than one imposes on other disciplines. To design a bridge that will bear its load, the engineer must, at least implicitly, rely on principles of physics that underlie the choices he makes. In learning those principles, he may consider hypothetical situations far removed from the details that he cannot ignore once he is in the field of design and construction. To choose the right action in a morally troubling situation, one must rely, at least implicitly, on principles of value that underlie the choices one makes. In learning those principles, one may have to consider hypothetical situations far removed from the details that one cannot ignore once one confronts the field of action.

We have journeyed far from that field in this chapter and have had a substantial dose of theoretical considerations. It is not yet clear whether these considerations can have any helpful bearing on the practical choices that are faced by physicians, patients, and others who are concerned about issues in health care. If an understanding of moral philosophy can be of some use in the face of such problems, it remains to be seen how. That question cannot be ignored, and we shall now move closer toward it by returning to some issues in clinical medicine.

6

The Impossibility of Value-Free Medicine

EACH NEW PHYSICIAN is faced with a complicated, often confusing array of decisions about what sort of physician to become. There are two sides to the question—not wholly separable, but distinguishable. One is the question of what the individual is most attracted to as an ideal professional life: Is it a life of medical research, advancing the frontiers; is it neurosurgery, with its high-risk, high-gain intensity; is it the more structured life of the radiologist, who can typically avoid the stress of midnight emergencies every few days; is it the glamour and intellectual dazzle of Park Avenue psychiatry or perhaps the satisfactions of a general practice bringing medical care to a low-income community that previously was isolated from access to good primary care? The other side is the question of what the world needs: Park Avenue may have enough psychiatrists; radiology may be saturated in a way in which geriatric medicine is unlikely ever to be; and the need for rural physicians may be largely unmet. So each medical student faces the prospect of trying to fashion a match between those career paths that constitute the stuff of fondest fantasy and those that give the outside world something it wants and is willing to pay for.

The lucky ones find a good fit easily; for others it is a lifelong struggle. However the choice is made, it will reflect the extent to which the individual is motivated by such factors as income opportunity, on the one hand, and a desire to serve those in need, on the other. Such a choice, and the way in which it is made, will reflect the basic values of the physician at a level that is concerned not so much with what to do in a particular situation as with what sort of person to be over the long run. To a lesser degree, the same sort of reflection of values will occur in the choice of the context of practice—whether it is to be in a health maintenance organization, a poverty clinic, a carriage trade office in the suburbs, or some other setting. Finally, the way in which the practice is structured—are the offices to be posh, the patients granted credit, the staff provided with good employee benefits?—will be determined in large measure not only by the prevailing conventions of organizing a medical practice, not by market conditions alone, but by the tastes and values of the physician whose practice it is, including that physician's sense of how it is appropriate to deal with other human beings.

It would be hard to dispute the claim that these choices are shaped in part by the values of the physician whose choices they are. Nor is it likely that anyone would object to the fact that values play such a role. In medicine, as elsewhere, how one chooses to lead one's life is largely one's right to choose as one will. And whereas we might be moved to praise the young physician who dedicates himself to rural family practice because of a commitment to social justice, we are not thereby denigrating those who are doing cardiac surgery in the metropolis. We might wish for a social policy that would lead a larger number of physicians to choose to help the disadvantaged populations, but we are not likely on that account alone to scorn the physician who pursues a dedication to a somewhat esoteric corner of medical research. Further, if we find that a physician is a mean-spirited, autocratic, unsympathetic employer, we will rightly think ill of the physician for that—not because we believe that the physician's values have no place in shaping professional behavior, but because we have contempt for the values that are manifested in the behavior we discover.

At the level of specific clinical decisions, the situation looks radically different. If a patient with a clearly broken hand enters the office of an orthopedic surgeon, we expect the response to be based solely on the medical possibilities of repairing the hand. (Assume that there are no special problems about payment, simultaneous emergencies competing for the physician's attention, or other extraneous grounds for taking exception to the claim.) The physician in this situation is free to have any sort of attitude at all toward the patient—repugnance, contempt, dislike, even loathing—so long as those attitudes remain private and do not influence the response to medical need. The hand is broken; the physician can repair the hand; therefore the physician must repair the hand—as well as possible—without regard to personal values that might lead the physician to think ill of the patient or of the patient's values. For instance, the physician may believe that work is crucial to good character, and the patient may be a bum who, although employable, prefers being on the dole; or the physician may be a devout believer in a religion the most effective public critic of which is the patient. It doesn't matter; the physician's personal, nonmedical values have no place here as an influence on medical decisions. That is what I mean here by the claim that clinical decisions should be value-free.

To sharpen the point, imagine the following dialogue. The physician enters, sees the patient, and speaks.

> "That's a pretty bad break you've got there. Here, let me have a closer look."
> "Can you fix it all right? Will it heal properly?"
> "Oh, I think it could be fixed; I've read the X rays, and I don't see any reason why it couldn't be fixed. But first, just what did you have in mind to do with it, Mr. . . . uh . . . ?"
> "Stern. Isaac Stern. I use it in my work."
> "Isaac Stern, the violinist?"
> "No, he's a distant relative. I'm Isaac Stern, the pickpocket."
> "Oh, I see. Well, sorry, we don't do pickpocket hands here. Nurse, show Mr. Stern out."

In this episode the physician has values that we might endorse—fine violinists are a benefit to society, pickpockets are not, and the general welfare might even be best served if the pickpocket were not properly treated—but we do not believe that it is proper for the physician to decide whether to set the broken bones on the basis of his own attitude toward what will be done with the hand after it heals. To do so is to import nonmedical values illegitimately into the practice of medicine and thereby to turn medical practice into an instrument for the furtherance of nonmedical aspects of social policy. That is a betrayal of the physician's obligations to cure and to heal and a betrayal of the trust that is bestowed in the granting of the license to practice medicine. The physician may condemn the pickpocket on moral grounds, but he must set the hand nonetheless.

A second example will be useful. A woman enters a gynecological clinic with a surgically correctable blockage of the fallopian tubes. She has been referred by an *in vitro* fertilization program on the grounds that her condition is surgically correctable and she is therefore not eligible as a candidate for IVF. The surgeon examines her, decides that her condition can be corrected, and then inquires:

> "Ms. Mammawollen, you understand that if you have this surgery, you will be able to become pregnant in the normal way?"
> "Oh, yes. That's why I want the operation. So I can have a child."
> "Are you married, Ms. M.?"
> "No, not yet."
> "Then with whom will you have a child?"

"I do have a boyfriend. If it works out, I think we may get married in a year or so."

"But we really don't know anything about him. Perhaps he is an unsuitable father. Or perhaps you won't actually marry him. Then there's no telling who you will be with next. I'm afraid we can't authorize the corrective surgery yet. We'll have to investigate your case. If we decide that it is a good thing for you to be able to get pregnant, we will do the operation. But if we are not confident that you will bring a wanted child into a wholesome and nurturing environment, then I think we'd best leave you as you are."

Here, too, we are appalled at the hypothetical physician's attempt to use the provision or denial of medical skills as an instrument for the furtherance of his personal values—and it does not help if we are in sympathy with those values, for what offends is not merely, or not at all, the values themselves but the way in which they are allowed to distort decisions that should be made solely on medical grounds. Again, at the level of clinical practice, medicine should be value-free in the sense that the personal values of the physician should not distort the making of medical decisions.

The examples we have just considered are fiction, toy examples invented to make a point. But the next case is fact. At a major university medical center there is a human fertility clinic; among the services it provides are genetic counseling, fertility testing, artificial insemination, and drug therapy. The process of obtaining artificial insemination involves a number of steps: The applicant's husband is tested to verify sterility, there is psychological counseling to ensure that the couple understands well what is involved in having a child by means of artificial insemination, and only then does treatment proceed. (I refer here to AID, artificial insemination with sperm from a donor—that is, someone other than the husband. Usually, it is not literally donated but is sold to the clinic, often by medical students who are convenient to the clinic, bright, in good health, and in need of extra income. There are also cases where, for special reasons, a woman is inseminated artificially with sperm donated by her husband; this is sometimes done in conjunction with sperm separation techniques that purport—controversially—to be able to increase the odds of having a child of a preselected sex.)

A psychiatrist at the clinic, also trained in gynecology, was involved in interviewing and counseling applicants for AID. Often couples come in together, but in this case a woman came alone. Early in the interview the physician asked her whether her husband had been tested to confirm sterility; she replied, to his surprise, "I don't have a husband."

Today that reply might be less startling; a few years ago, at the time of these events, it was new in the experience of the physician. Taken aback, he said, "I'm not quite sure what to say here. I haven't seen a case of this kind come up before, and I'm just not sure what our clinic's policy would be on inseminating an unmarried woman."

"I'm not actually—I don't consider myself—an unmarried woman," she responded. And as the psychiatrist masked his dismay as well as he could, she went on to explain that she considered herself to be married in a stable, long-term lesbian relationship. She and her partner had decided that they wanted a child and that she would bear it. She knew, she said, that she could get herself pregnant in the usual way, but that would involve both a violation of her personal integrity as a committed lesbian and a shameful and deceptive use of some man as an instrument in pursuit of her purposes. Her only honorable course, she pointed out, was AID. The physician's dismay was of a fairly sophisticated sort. At once he knew that any position he took bore risks. If he indicated approval, he might encounter a maelstrom of opposition from his peers in the clinic, some of whom were certain to disapprove of the idea of the clinic's being complicit in such an undertaking. And if he indicated opposition or refusal, for all he knew he might be slapped with some sort of suit on the ground of making discriminatory judgments. There was federal funding in the clinic, and he was unsure just what the limits of the clinic's rights of refusal were. More importantly, he wanted to respond in the way that was right on the merits of the case, but not having thought about such cases at all, he was entirely uncertain what the merits of the case were. Wisely he decided that he needed time to investigate the case and discuss it with others, and he therefore asked the patient to return the following week with her partner to discuss the situation, this being the normal procedure with a typical couple. (It was between these two appointments that I met the physician and heard about the case.)

I have often described this case to classes and audiences, essentially as I have recounted it now. And the question I then ask is whether or not in the final analysis the woman's application should be approved or refused. Always there is dispute; often the response is fairly evenly divided; typically it is heated. You can repeat the exercise easily; gather some friends, present the case, and ask them what their vote would be. But it is the next step that is most important—the provision of the reasons that justify the position that one takes. The positions, and the supporting reasons for them, run the gamut from refusal based on the most virulent sort of opposition to homosexuality to approval based on the view that no consideration is relevant except the clinic's technical ability to provide the service as requested. Neither of these views had any appeal to the physician who faced the case. But most of the other reasons that I have heard people offer on either side did occur to him. And the dialogue that follows can therefore be seen as a recapitulation of the deliberations that raced through his mind as he searched for that initial response.

A: The physician's obligation is to serve the patient. It's as simple as that. The patient has a need that the clinic can meet, so the answer has to be yes. Nothing else bears on the case. He's got no right to refuse just because her family situation is one that he sees as odd or unusual or anything else.

B: But giving her AID isn't providing medical treatment to a patient. The physician has no obligation to her, and saying yes wouldn't cure any problem or disease she's got. She's just asking the physician to help her get something she wants, and under the circumstances it's a pretty weird desire at that. Maybe she wants a yacht, too. But the physician has no responsibility to cater to her desires just because it is in the power of the clinic to do it. The AID program was set up as a service to infertile married couples, and there's no reason to extend it to a case like this. He should just say no.

A: But the AID isn't just one thing this woman desires. It's a desire that can be met by a service that this clinic is in the business of providing. The question of cure has nothing to do with it; that's as irrelevant in this case as it is in the case of the normal woman in a normal marriage who just has a sterile husband. Nothing gets cured there either. If the clinic will help satisfy the desire for a child in the one case, how can it refuse in the other? There are no good grounds to say no.

B: There are if you think of the child. And you must think of the child. The physician doesn't have to be complicit in bringing a child into an environment like that. Just think of the burdens on that kid—no father and, if that isn't bad enough, somewhere between one and two mothers, depending on how you count. What does he tell the other kids? What kind of model for male-female relationships does he grow up with? If it is a girl, what chance does she have for normal heterosexual development? If it's a boy, what kind of psychological environment are a couple of man-haters going to give him? The physician should say no for the sake of the child, and he's got every right to do so.

A: But you don't know that it would be like that at all. What evidence is there that two women can't raise a child well? Maybe these two can't, and maybe they can. Do you really have a good basis for deciding they can't, or is it just a lot of conventional prejudice that's showing? Because unless you can really make a case that these women would be bad parents, I don't see how you can deny them the chance.

B: Maybe there isn't what you would call hard data. There just aren't enough cases of the right kind about which enough is known. But if you think about it, you can't help seeing that it isn't a wholesome environment. I mean, think about what adoption agencies do. They have a tremendous amount of experience. They aren't going to place a kid in a home like that. They take the question of parental suitability very seriously, and it is well known how hard it can be to get an adoptive child. They know what they are doing, and they would surely vote no on this one.

A: In the first place, adoption agencies are ridiculous. If you aren't some sort of paradigm of wage-earning, churchgoing, middle-class solid citizen, they write you off, no matter how full of love and good sense you are. But if you meet the tests on their little checklists, then it's fine, even if you're really a sleazy tyrant beneath the veneer of respectability. But that isn't even the point. Those agencies are finding homes for kids that already exist. So they can be fussy, especially when they're in a good market situation. But they don't go around saying who can and who can't have kids in the first place. Even if they're right in their views about parental suitability, they don't propose to extend their standards to determine who can have children on their own. I'm not so sure that they would say no for this case, but even if they would, that has nothing to do with the fact that the physician should say yes.

B: But is that right? Or does the argument cut the other way, maybe. There isn't anything more important than the quality of the job that parents do. And you're right, the clinic isn't in the business of curing medical problems. It provides a service that people want, and in that way maybe it is more like a social service agency. Perhaps it should act more like one and start considering parental suitability for all applicants. The lesson of this case may be that the clinic has been entirely too superficial in screening cases. If an applicant is married to a sterile man but is also a drug-addicted prostitute, the clinic should recognize that there's no parental suitability there either and should turn that case down as well.

A: That's wrong. It's wrong on two different grounds. First, it's a start down the path to social control of the worst sort. The clinic judges who gets to have children and who doesn't! But why limit that kind of screening just to the cases that need a fertility clinic? Surely most of the worst parents are physically normal and would never come near the clinic. So if you want to screen to protect potential kids against being born into bad families by preventing their being born at all, you have to screen more broadly. You have to have licenses for people to reproduce. Anybody who gets pregnant without a license is a criminal unless there is an immediate abortion. Maybe only the people with college degrees get to have kids, or the number you get to have depends upon your rank or your politics. That kind of thinking would tear the society apart. But anyway, there's the second reason, and that's much simpler. Everybody has the right to reproduce. To say no is to deny the woman's autonomy with respect to one of the most basic and personal choices that anyone can make.

B: But the point is that most people are not patients at the clinic—you just said so yourself. And that defeats your scare tactic argument about fascism. I'm not proposing anything about a general social policy. I'm talking about how the clinic should respond to the cases that do come to it. They will always be a small minority of the population. I'm suggesting not that the clinic should go out making judgments about the society at large, but that in facing the cases that come to it, it should take all the factors into account, including the interests of the potential children, and then it should have the courage to say no when it concludes that it is a bad situation for a child. It isn't a question of the clinic's deciding what other people do; it *is* a question of the clinic's deciding what the clinic will do. And that is a question of rights, too. A physician should have the right to refuse to do something he judges to be wrong. A devout Catholic physician doesn't have to do abortions, and shouldn't have to—everybody agrees to that on all sides of the abortion debate—and neither should any physician have to inseminate a woman who he's convinced won't be able to provide a decent home for a child.

A: So now we're back to where we started. Even if the physician is convinced a woman won't provide a decent home, what makes that opinion so important? Do they learn in medical school how to test for decent motherhood? That's nothing more than making the physician a moral arbiter without any real basis of expertise. One physician might be homophobic, and the next might be a lesbian herself; but the personal values of the physician have to get set aside, and the nonmedical beliefs do also. The physicians should do what they are trained to do, and that is to provide the services that will help their patients, without trying to fit it all into a larger judgment about the whole social order.

This debate could go on at length, but it is not my intention to pursue it. For the point is not to decide whether the final decision should be to inseminate the woman. It is instead to learn something from the uncertainty that this case generates.

A great many issues arose in the brief debate that represented the physician's uncertainties about how to respond. (If we had pursued the debate, more would likely have arisen.) These issues included the question of the proper function of medical services; the interests of the potential child; the difference between the interests of the actual people who are the subjects of adoption agency activities and the potential, but not actual, people who are the subjects of fertility clinic activities; the extent and nature of the right to reproduce; the possibility of establishing criteria for parental suitability; the right of the providers of medical services to refuse treatment and the question of what it takes to justify such refusal; and the competence of the physician or other clinic staff to make decisions that go beyond the medical factors in the case.

Each of these issues invites extended debate and examination, but extended debate and examination are a luxury that can rarely be afforded in the context of a clinical decision. Indeed, this case is unusual in that it provided the physician an opportunity to defer response for a week, making it possible for him to discuss the case with a variety of people whose advice he could incorporate, as he saw fit, into the decision he finally made. More often, morally challenging situations in medicine require that some decision be made with substantial speed—rarely in a matter of moments, but more commonly on the order of hours or days than on the order of weeks. In such situations, physicians and patients may be well served by having thought about ethical conflict in advance.

The factors that bear on a case like this are of diverse kinds. Some are matters of fact, such as what will actually happen to the child if the woman is inseminated and what the law requires or allows the clinic to do. Other factors are matters of social policy, such as the nature and extent of the right to reproduce. (Would a pregnant woman have a right to take drugs that would cause her child to be a dwarf in order to fulfill a lifelong ambition to be the mother of a circus performer? I ask the question to show that we do believe there should be some limits on the rights of reproduction.) Still other factors are matters neither of empirical fact nor of social policy, but of judgment and value, such as the questions of what counts as parental suitability or how much the potential interests of the possible child should count, as against the actual interests of the actual woman who wants to have a child. Despite these differences in kind among the various factors that arise in the debate, however, one question must be faced with respect to each of them—the question of whether that factor is relevant to the decision at all.

If one believes that a pure consequentialism such as classical act utilitarianism is the correct guide to action, all the factors that are raised will be seen as relevant to the extent that they have bearing on what the consequences of treatment and of refusal would be. In particular, if the child *would* be likely to have an unfortunate childhood, that factor would have to be taken into account. Of course, in such a view, that is because such factors should always be taken into account; there is nothing about this situation that makes the difference. This is not to say that a rule utilitarian would have to believe that decisions about AID should be based on considerations of parental suitability. Instead, a utilitarian might argue that the greatest good for the greatest number will be produced in the long run if considerations of parental suitability are generally not taken into account. But the empirical facts about what will happen in any particular case must always be recognized as *relevant* by the act utilitarian;

this might be the one unanticipated case that requires modifying the general policy.

The question of the physician's obligations will be considered in a parallel way. To the extent that honoring an obligation serves the general interest, the utilitarian will say the physician must honor that obligation—but not otherwise. Or the rule utilitarian could argue that it serves the general welfare best for physicians always to honor their obligations, but the holder of such a view would still have to consider in any particular case whether, on the basis of the empirical facts, the particular features of the case justify modification of the general rule about obligations.

Utilitarianism is thus future-oriented; it bases the judgment about what is right to do on considerations of what consequences will follow in the future from each of the various actions under consideration. But it is possible to argue against the utilitarian position, holding that what one ought to do depends more on what has happened in the past or on what is true in the present than on what will happen in the future. If, for example, the clinic has promised its financial backers to provide AID to any applicant who is medically qualified to receive it, there is an obligation based on that past occurrence to approve the application that is pending, no matter what the consequences of such approval might be. It could then be argued that although the financial backers did not have this sort of case in mind and would willingly change the policy for the future, in the present circumstances there is no just basis for refusal. Or one could argue that the woman's right to reproduce is not tempered by any considerations of what the consequences will be if she exercises that right. (This would not by itself entail that the clinic has an obligation to assist her in the exercise of that right. At most, it would entail that the clinic has an obligation not to interfere with her exercise of that right.)

Such critics of a utilitarian position would thus rule out as not relevant a number of the factors that for the utilitarian are central to the case. And in particular, one factor that would not count as morally relevant is the actual outcome for the mother and the child. If refusal results in misery for the woman or a subsequent sense of relief in retrospect that she narrowly averted a moral and personal disaster, or if approval results in the joyful raising of a happy and well-adjusted child or leads to a life of torment for both the mother and the child, these considerations depend on myriad other influences that come into play as the world unfolds and have no bearing on the original decision about what is right to do. For the nonconsequentialist, it isn't the consequences that count, but whether rights have been respected, obligations honored, promises kept. So before the physician who faces the decision can properly assess the factors we have mentioned and then take them into account, he must make a decision about what *sorts* of factors are the morally relevant ones. Only after concluding that a factor is of a sort that should have bearing on the decision can he proceed to give it its proper place in the deliberation. But that will be difficult unless he understands fairly well who, morally speaking, he is. Thus, just as it is important for physicians to be sensitive to the values of their patients, it is also important—and can be comparably difficult—for them to have a sensitive awareness of what their own values are.

Any decision in the case at hand will obviously be determined by a number of considerations, the assessment of which will itself be determined in part by the moral outlook of the physician who must make the decision. No response to this situation can be value-free, for even to decide to treat the woman solely on the ground that she is a medically qualified applicant is to endorse the controversial social policy that such cases should be considered solely on grounds of medical suitability—a position disputed by approximately half of each medical school class that I have asked to consider it.

But this case, it might be argued, provides no evidence that the practice of medicine, more generally, is value-laden. This case is loaded at the outset with the ingredients of ethical debate: sexual preferences, reproductive behavior, illegitimacy, technologically aided conception, parental suitability. This is surely a case the mere appearance of which could reasonably be viewed by the physician as a moral disaster—in the sense that being fraught with conflict, it imposes on him an inescapable necessity of doing something that will provide, at best, the grounds for deep misgivings. Of course, medical education provides no training that will help in a case like this, but this case is just a bit of bad moral luck; one can expect such episodes to be rare enough in the practice of medicine that it is an error to agonize over their apparent intractability. There are two replies to this response, a response I see as self-indulgently comforting. First, it overestimates the rarity of moral conflict. Secondly, it overestimates the importance of rarity.

The case we have just considered does present ethical conflict in a highly visible way. But ethically loaded decisions are part and parcel of medical practice. They arise in the case of the comatose emergency patient who can be resuscitated but who is highly likely to have severe brain damage if revived. They arise in the physician's way of handling his own chronic tardiness. They arise in the use of pain-killing drugs; in the judgments that are made about patient education, informed consent, and patient autonomy; and even in the choice of language that communicates bad news to patients. In several chapters we have seen cases that illustrate how the making of medical decisions depends on considerations of value as well as on medical factors. The ideal of filtering out the judgmental aspects of such decisions is unrealistic.

Physicians can achieve partial success at limiting their judgments to the areas within which they have expertise, but partial success is all that it will ever be. For the business of medicine is essentially the minding of other people's business, albeit in a limited way. So the physician cannot escape moral dilemmas by deciding to mind his own business— medical decision—while leaving to others the responsibility of minding theirs. Medicine is by its nature intrusive in the lives of its consumers; the providers therefore cannot escape the fact that there are ethical dimensions of nearly all they do. Even when a situation seems wholly uncontroversial—a bandage for a scraped knee or an aspirin for a sore throat— the manner in which the case is handled has ethical underpinnings and overtones. And even to do the obvious, uncontroversial thing is to make a choice that affirms and endorses the values that underlie that conventional response. So taking comfort in the prospect of escape from ethical issues on grounds of statistical infrequency provides a thin refuge indeed.

More important, the rarity of ethical dilemmas of a serious sort— whatever the degree of that rarity—should also be of limited comfort. We do not consider a man honest merely because he is mainly honest, stealing only twice a year or only from one corporation. We do not consider a woman courageous although she falters only rarely, when she faces danger. A man is not gentle who beats his wife or children only from time to time, nor is she kindly who is intermittently cruel. Morality is more demanding than that. Even if one were rarely challenged by difficult situations, it would be nonetheless true that the measure of one's character would still depend largely on the way one rose to the occasion when challenge did occur.

The problem of just how demanding the requirements of moral integrity really are is a central one for moral theory. Few would argue in favor of a position so austere as to judge one a moral failure for having made moral errors from time to time. Perfection is elusive in every sphere of life, and just as it is inevitable that physicians will make medical mistakes, provided only that they practice medicine, so, too, will one surely make moral errors, doing what is wrong from time to time, so long as one lives and acts. What is less clear is how closely to moral perfection one should approximate in one's objectives or in the standard one uses for judging oneself. A surgeon must take every surgical error seriously but must not be crippled by discouragement at having erred. Rather, the ability to accept and learn from one's mistakes is a necessary part of success in becoming a surgeon. Similarly, a commitment to acting in an ethical way requires that one be able to accept, learn from, and transcend one's own moral errors and failings. But just how good must one be?

Classical utilitarianism holds that one must act always so as to produce the greatest happiness for the greatest number. Taken literally, this theory seems to require saintliness. For, when we are given almost any action performed in the course of normal everyday life, there seems to be something else one could have chosen to do that would have been more productive of total human happiness. Are you reading a book, mildly enjoying it? You could be working as a volunteer, comforting the dying in a hospital. Did you take an evening off to relax at a movie? You could have been working to relieve hunger among the poor. So an additional problem with utilitarianism is that it seems so demanding as to be incompatible with what we are inclined, even on reflection, to believe is morally required of us.

Other moral theories face similar difficulties, seeming to hold us to standards that are beyond the psychological reach even of people who are generally thought of as exemplars of decency. This may account in part for the appeal that some people find in the moral views that seem (for they are not explicit) to inform Nozick's radical political libertarianism. If a theory asks of you only that you refrain from violating the rights of others, it is relatively easy to comply—easy, at least, compared with what is required by a moral theory that asks us to respect the rights of others and *also* to act in the interests of their welfare. Libertarianism (as a moral theory, not merely as a viewpoint on political organization) forbids us to violate another person's right to life, for example, but places no burden on us to care about it or to make any effort to sustain it— except as we are committed by contract or other special obligations to do so. (The moral libertarian, of course, *allows* us to be moved to help another by charitable inclinations but cannot consistently require us to do so.) Utilitarianism, on the other hand, is an activist morality, charging us to value the interests of others as we do our own. So the question of how demanding of us a moral theory may properly be turns out to be inseparable from the question of which moral theory most properly merits acceptance.

A moral theory, to be plausible at all, must help us distinguish, from among the things we *might* do, the one (or more) which is right. If a theory about morality—or even a single moral guideline or principle— asks of us that we do what is not possible for us to do, then it can have no bearing on our choices and becomes irrelevant to human behavior.

Nor will a theory that fails to distinguish one choice from another among those we face be acceptable; this is the primary failing of what has been called the ethics of love—the theory that admonishes us to do the loving thing without providing us with any way of identifying the one that merits that honorific description.[1] But even theories that seem quite clear in the direction they provide will leave us with substantial uncertainty. Utilitarianism, for example, in calling for the act that maximizes happiness, confronts us with the task of making what are sometimes exquisitely difficult assessments of what the consequences of the various options before us will be. This is why, even for the untempered utilitarian, the case of the woman seeking AID is a very difficult one to assess. Still, the utilitarian has a clear sense of what the relevant factors are, and the theory thus shapes and directs moral inquiry for him. And the proponent of an ethics of love would presumably have the moral inquiry shaped in a different way, perhaps with a focus on motivation rather than on outcomes.

If we are given that a moral theory, even when it cannot readily identify what one ought to do, can nonetheless direct one's further explorations by separating out the relevant from the irrelevant considerations, and are given that the practice of medicine involves frequent encounters with the need to make decisions about morally troubling cases, it follows that it would be useful for physicians to have some definitive indication of what the correct moral theory is. But questions of value seem to be precisely those about which we find the greatest dispute, and when we move from a particular disputed case or question of policy to the more basic foundations of moral judgment, we find that the dispute goes right along with us. Controversy about moral matters swirls around us whenever we lift our heads from the daily routine long enough to reflect for even a moment about the moral dilemmas we face. But is the situation hopeless? Can moral philosophy help, or is one in the end cast back entirely on one's own hunches about what to do? And if there is some help to be found, how is that compatible with the diversity of values that we encounter?

7

Resolving Moral Conflict: The Challenge

IT IS TIME TO ASK whether and to what extent the moral problems in medicine and health policy can be solved and whether moral philosophy can contribute in any useful way to such solutions as are possible. These are no idle queries; their answers are in dispute both among medical practitioners and among philosophers, some of whom despair of finding any help in philosophical speculations, in view of the widespread disagreement about values at every level of debate. We live in a secular, pluralistic age, some have argued, adrift in a sea of moral conflict without any dominant moral direction to guide us toward solutions to the tragic crises that we face. The price we have paid for moral diversity is moral chaos—so the argument goes.

It was not always so. There have been times and circumstances in which a sense of moral clarity prevailed, when a single moral outlook was dominant and provided a uniform perspective for judging actions and facing decisions. Moral error and moral conflict did not engender constant dispute. Heretics were simply burned, perhaps, or gangsters hanged from the gallows. Or the agent who faced a moral dilemma could take it to an expert for good counsel or even arbitration. For example, one of the traditional functions of the village rabbi was as judge in moral matters, and individuals in dilemma as well as parties in dispute would come to the rabbi in search of a resolution of the quandary or dispute. A common allegiance to mutually accepted values provided the conceptual background for the resolutions they obtained. Similar phenomena occur in other closely knit communities with a shared perspective both on basic values and on the methods and principles for resolving particular conflicts in terms of those basic values. But for us, no such unity of outlook exists.

Some people have seen this circumstance as an indication of moral decay or as a fall from grace, lamenting the loss of a unified moral outlook precisely because such an outlook makes possible and legitimate the definitive resolution of moral conflicts. But it is a different view of the matter that I shall advocate here, arguing that although definitive resolution of moral problems is indeed out of reach, it is an error to despair of being able to clarify moral problems in a way that can help resolve them.

A biologist—one of a group of science and engineering professors who came together for a month of intensive study of moral philosophy one recent summer—listened attentively to three weeks of lectures, read the relevant literature with care, participated vigorously in the discussions, and, at the end of the third week, plaintively announced, "The deeper I get into this, the clearer it seems that it doesn't get better; it only gets worse." It provides little comfort to learn that a problem you thought was distressingly complex is actually more complex than you thought. But the case for moral philosophy does not rest on the enterprise's provid-ing comfort. The objective, rather, is twofold. One is the achievement of a higher level of understanding of moral judgment and moral reason-ing, entirely apart from any benefit that it may yield in the face of practical decisions. The other is to help us make moral decisions that are better, not necessarily easier, than those we would make with lesser understand-ing. It is this second objective that is our present concern; judged in terms of it, moral philosophy has earned a passing grade.

To defend that claim, I must first discuss pluralism, closure, and judg-ment. Pluralism in respect to values is the coexistence of different beliefs about the nature and source of value. When it was generally believed that right action was action that conformed to the will of God, and when that belief was powerfully enough entrenched to be able to silence dissenting viewpoints before they could establish any substantial following, there was moral hegemony, not pluralism. It does not matter that there was dispute about how to tell what conformed to the mysterious divine will, nor does it matter that some actions prompted by that moral outlook were atrocities. The fact remains that there flourished a moral perspective that for an extended period had no serious competition within the culture that sustained it. But now, despite the fact that some people yearn for such simpler times, we have utilitarians, Kantians, moral relativists, "situation ethicists," religious fundamentalists, secular humanists, libertarians, and a host of folks who espouse a variety of homespun views that range over the thoughtful, the vague, the inconsistent, and the incoherent. And the climate of the times suggests that we should respect them all, almost as if they were matters of taste with respect to which no objections could be truly telling. It is this climate of tolerance, combined with the pluralism of moral outlooks, that gives rise to the sense that moral arguments are impossible to resolve on reasonable grounds.

Closure is the resolution of an argument or debate, as opposed to its mere termination. That is, a dispute or disagreement can end because one party has more power and can impose a decision, because one party simply tires of the argument and goes away, or in a variety of other ways that do not involve the disputants' coming to agreement on the issue or even agreeing to accept a single outcome. But sometimes a dispute ends because the parties to it have worked through the issue to a point of common understanding; the debate is closed because the disagreement is dispelled. It is that sort of closure that seems most elusive in the context of moral pluralism, and it is that sort of closure that I want to discuss.

Judgment is perhaps the hardest of these notions to characterize. Some decisions can be made in accordance with procedures that specify precisely how the decision should vary with the circumstances. A simple example is the behavior of drivers approaching a traffic signal. If the light is red, the driver should stop; if it is green, the driver should continue on. The driver simply follows the rules. Of course, sometimes the rules that govern a procedure are very complex. Finding a break in the circuit of a complicated piece of electronic equipment, for example, can be challenging and time-consuming despite the fact that there are rules that specify, step by step, how one is to proceed until the break is found. Some portions of mathematics, too, provide illustrations. A problem in arithmetic can be trivial, compared with a complicated problem of calculus, but each is solvable in accordance with a procedure that can be specified on a step-by-step basis. (Such procedures are called decision procedures or algorithms.) But not all decisions can be made in accordance with a procedure that is guaranteed to yield the desired result if followed correctly. Instead, a person faced with a decision must often depend on some elusive combination of taste, hunch, intuition, and skill of a sort that is impossible to characterize rigorously.

A few examples should illustrate the point. One can explain with precision the rules for writing a sonnet. Following those rules will guarantee that one will produce a sonnet, but not that the sonnet will be any good. There are no rules for that; creative ability is not a matter of rule following. But it isn't only in matters of art in the literal sense that quality of performance depends on something that is never quite captured by the rules. In every walk of personal and professional life there is a place for judgment. The scientist who time after time pursues a fruitful line of research, while others are grinding away at problems that are pedestrian or dead ends, is admired as having a "good nose" for what is important in the discipline. That sense of what is important may be passed on through apprenticeship to the better students, but it has never been characterized in any systematic way that would lead to a set of instructions for success. The distinguished chef seems able to produce what cannot be duplicated even by one who follows the recipe precisely; the very precision is a constraint on the exercise of the skills that set the distinguished chef apart. The political speechwriter, the advertising executive, the film editor, the lawyer arguing before a jury, the teacher communicating effectively with a class, the interviewer getting a recalcitrant subject to open up, the architect matching a floor plan to a client's needs, the business executive assessing the wisdom of expansion into a new territory, the academic administrator exercising leadership among the faculty, and innumerable others all are engaged in activities that can be done well or badly but that cannot be directed by an algorithm for success. Rather, they call for the agent to integrate the accumulated evidence, from all quarters, that is relevant to the performance of such tasks and then to make a decision that is constrained, but not wholly determined, by the codified wisdom of the discipline in question. Violating such codified wisdom will likely ensure failure, but abiding by it will never be a guarantee of success, for in these undertakings such rules as exist are at best necessary conditions for doing well, not sufficient conditions for success. The gap between the codified understanding of how to do a thing well and the action that one takes in doing it is closed by the exercise of judgment.

There are rules, theories, guidelines, and compendiums of advice for scientists, journalists, lawyers, teachers, and all the rest. And in each of these areas there are those who cope, those who fail, and those who excel. What separates them from one another is largely the quality of judgment they exercise in pursuit of their objectives. So, too, there are good and evil people. The position for which I will argue is that here, too, what separates them one from the other is not adherence to an algorithm for moral behavior but is largely the quality of judgment they exercise in the face of ethically difficult choices.

Decisions can be difficult to make for many different reasons. One can need facts that are not available or are difficult or costly to obtain. (Shall I carry the umbrella? I'd know if I knew the odds of rain. Shall I drill for oil here? We can explore the site, but even that is expensive. Shall I use this drug? There's no way to predict what effect it will have on this patient, although it has helped some others who are in some ways similar.)

Or one might be immobilized by anxiety or by uncertainty about how to compare the relative merits of a high-risk, high-gain choice and a low-risk, low-gain choice. (Shall I bet on the favorite or the long shot?) Such problems of decision can sometimes have ethical aspects, but they are not cases in which the primary source of dilemma is uncertainty about the moral aspects of the situation.

In other cases, however, a choice can be hard because of the conflict in values that it involves. It is important here to be clear about what sort of conflict this is. I am not concerned with the utilitarian's uncertainty about what to do when it is unclear which action will produce the best consequences, for that is a factual uncertainty, resolvable to the extent that empirical evidence can illuminate what effects will flow from what causes. Nor am I concerned with a Rawlsian's uncertainty about whether a particular deviation from equality will accrue to the benefit of the least advantaged, for that, too, is a question of empirical fact. I am concerned, however, with the person who sees the attraction both in the Kantian adherence to obligations as strictly binding and in the utilitarian commitment to maximizing happiness and who is torn between those two attractions in facing a situation in which an obligation can be met only at a substantial cost in terms of happiness. This might be the plight, for example, of a physician who has promised to tell the truth to a patient and who then comes to believe that doing so will be detrimental to the patient's prospects for recovery. It is problems such as these that are at issue, in which the primary uncertainty is about what is right, rather than about what is likely or possible.

In a particularly insightful essay on "The Fragmentation of Value," Thomas Nagel has argued persuasively that conflict and uncertainty of this sort result inevitably from the fact that the sources of value are diverse.[1] Human beings, he writes, are capable of viewing the world from various points of view, including the perspective of an individual considering his own interests and the development of his own life, of a person concerned with his relationships to other people, of a person transcending the particularities of his own existence to view the world with an impersonal interest in what is best for people generally, and in other ways as well. These different perspectives give rise to values of different kinds—the relational viewpoint underlies our concern with rights and obligations, the impersonal viewpoint yields a concern with social utility, and so on. Since each of these ways of viewing the world has legitimacy, there is no justifiable way to elevate one to a position of dominance, and thus, we will frequently face situations in which our values pull us simultaneously in different directions. For the complexity that allows us to adopt these different perspectives also requires us to do so. Pluralism, Nagel would likely agree, results not merely from the differences between different persons when they think about matters of value but, perhaps more basically, is a feature of the attitude toward values that each of us has.

If pluralism with respect to values is a feature not merely of groups of people but of the outlook of individuals also, the possibilities for closure in the face of moral dilemmas may seem slender. In the case of the woman requesting artificial insemination, we considered a debate that was truncated with no indication that closure was in prospect. But in the case of the elderly woman dying in the hospital, whose son persuaded the physician to modify the medical orders, there was a resolution that should count as closure. That was not a difficult case, for no deep conflict of values was involved in it. Instead, the physician was merely unaware of the way in which his assumptions about value were directing his choices at the level of clinical decisions. Once he understood what was happening, his commitment to patient autonomy as well as to beneficence led him to agree with the son about what should be done. A more difficult situation is that in which various physicians disagreed about whether or not to sustain life because they had different reasons for seeing life as valuable.

There is temptation in the face of such conflicts to hope for solutions in an appeal to moral rules. This hope can assume ambitious proportions. I once had a student who had majored in computer science before entering medical school. His vision was of a computer-based algorithm for the resolution of the moral problems in clinical practice. Each ethically troubling problem that had occurred would be analyzed, the relevant considerations assessed, the decision recorded, the outcome documented, and the whole fed into the computer's memory. When enough cases of a particular kind had occurred, some generalizations about their handling could be inferred; that, too, could become part of the data base. Once the system was established, it would be possible to rely on it for the solutions to new cases as they arose. It was to be, I conjectured to his mild discomfort, a space-age technological imitation of the village rabbi. For example, had the system been in place when the lesbian requested insemination, the physician could have requested an immediate printout of information about relevant cases and considerations; he would thereby be guided to the proper solution for the case he faced.

Such a dream is fantasy, but not innocent fantasy. It diverts attention from the realities of ethical conflicts and the demands that they place on those who face them. Had the physician sat scanning the printout, he would probably have noticed that no case of the kind was yet on record.

But even if similar cases had been faced before, the physician would have had to decide whether they were sufficiently like the case in hand in the morally relevant respects for them to be considered as cases of the same sort. And if we assume that they were relevantly similar—and assume further, as is unlikely, that they had been handled in a uniform way—the question of whether or not this case ought to be handled as they had been would still remain. For the decision to follow a precedent is a substantive moral decision; there is always the option of judging the previous case to have been handled wrongly and of acting differently in the case at hand. No such judgment can be made or defeated by the computer. It can supply a wealth of factual data, much of which may indeed be useful to the physician who faces a difficult decision. But in the final analysis, the result will be only that the physician is better armed in facing the decision, not relieved of the burden of facing it. What the student had revealed was a far grander version, but a version all the same, of the avoidance behavior of the medical student who seeks relief from the rigors of moral thought in the refuge of acquisition of facts.

The appeal to moral rules fares little better. Consider the case of action aimed at terminating a life—perhaps of a minimally viable neonatal monstrosity, perhaps of a dying patient in intractable agony, perhaps of a fetus the abortion of which is contemplated. "Thou shalt not kill," reads the commandment, and nearly everyone assents. But almost no one believes it. Rather, nearly everyone believes that there are circumstances in which the taking of a life is justifiable. For many, the needs of national defense can provide the justification; for most, self-defense or defense of one's loved ones can count as grounds for waiver of the rule; and for some, the commitment of sufficiently serious crimes can warrant the taking of a life, even of someone who presents no continuing threat to anyone. It does not matter here what one sees as justification for taking a life, however; the point is that nearly everyone agrees that there are *some* justifications. The rule that one may not kill is thus reinterpreted; insofar as we accept it, we take it to mean that one must not kill *except with justification*. That is a much weaker rule, but it still has moral content. I can whistle a tune as I walk down the street, and I don't owe anyone a justification of my behavior. I am free to do it if I choose. But I am not comparably free to kill another person. This is not merely a point of law; if the laws against murder were repealed, it would still be morally unacceptable for me to kill another without reason. So what the commandment really means is essentially that if you kill someone, you'd better have a pretty good story about why, or else you are in trouble, morally as well as legally.

Now let us return to one of the disputed cases. Suppose we wonder whether the killing of a particular fetus is right or not, and we seek relief from the puzzlement by appealing to the rule that one should not kill. Since the rule bans killing except where it is justified, we cannot tell whether the rule prohibits the action we are considering unless we know first whether the contemplated killing *is* justified. But that is the very puzzle we faced in the first place. So the rule fails to help us decide about cases that raise doubts about whether a particular act of killing is justified. But those are the only cases that tempt us to seek help from the rule! We need not consult it, after all, to discover that it is unjustified to chop off a neighbor's head for playing the radio too loudly at night or that it is justified to shoot a man who is shooting at our children and who cannot be stopped any other way. So the rule seems to apply clearly where we don't need it and can gain no help from it, but where we are in doubt about whether an act of killing is justified or not, that very doubt makes the rule useless to us. Since moral rules typically have this character, there is little hope of dissolving ethical problems in general by invoking the appropriate moral rule. We are no more likely to escape from moral problems by reaching into a satchel of rules than we are by turning to a computer.

Alasdair MacIntyre, in an eloquent essay hidden in an esoteric volume, has recently presented a starkly pessimistic position about the prospects for resolution of moral conflict and about the possibility of moral philosophy's being of any practical service in the effort.[2] His views are more fully presented in his brilliant and important new book, *After Virtue*.[3] His arguments are worth considering in full; I cannot do justice to them here. But there need be no confusion about his conclusions, for he states them quite clearly. Referring to the morally troubling questions in medical practice, he says, "We have no rational method available for reaching a conclusion in these questions." Rejecting the possibility that this unhappy state is due either to the special character of these problems or to the general character of moral argument, he places the blame squarely on "the peculiar character of moral debate in our liberal, secular, pluralist culture." And he concludes:

What makes any protagonist's situation tragic is that he inevitably has to choose between wrong and wrong. It is with this in mind that I have spoken of the physician's moral dilemmas as tragic. The moral resources of his culture, of our own culture, offer no solution for him. What matters most in a period in which human life is tragic is to have the strength to resist false solutions. . . .

The medical profession ought not therefore to look for solutions to philosophical theorizing; what philosophy has to tell them is precisely why there are no solutions.[4]

I reject this characterization of what philosophy has to tell the medical profession. But I believe I understand how MacIntyre comes to hold it. If we accept the view that an adequate moral theory must enable us to resolve any moral dilemma, and if we then observe that there seems to be no moral theory that performs such a function, we can conclude that there is no adequate moral theory. It then follows that there is no moral theory adequate to resolve the physician's dilemmas in particular and, further, that physicians ought not look to moral philosophy for such solutions. If the absence of an adequate moral theory is due to our liberal, secular, pluralist culture, so be it; it is an absence all the same.

There is some evidence that MacIntyre holds such a view of moral philosophy. He speaks of "a morality adequate to guide a human life," argues that virtues and vices can be distinguished only against the background of an "over-all interpretation of human existence," and claims that our "fragmented" moral inheritance has left us "resourceless in the face of moral problems." I have a sense here of an attitude toward moral philosophy that reflects a quest for moral certainty, much as Descartes sought epistemological certainty. MacIntyre would have us believe that because we have no coherent, all-encompassing moral perspective, we are morally resourceless. But the quest for moral certainty makes no more sense than Descartes's quest. Rationality demands that we accept less than perfect evidence as being good enough to warrant belief—because there is no perfect evidence. Similarly, there is no perfect assurance of moral rectitude, and moral courage demands that we accept less than perfect moral reasoning as being good enough to warrant action. In ethics, as in epistemology, uncertainty can have its place, without undermining the enterprise in its entirety.

It will be instructive to consider how MacIntyre supports his claim of moral resourcelessness. We are given three pairs of arguments, each with plausible premises and inferences, and with mutually incompatible conclusions:

1(a).

> I cannot will that my mother should have had an abortion when she was
> pregnant with me, except perhaps if it had been certain that the embryo
> was dead or gravely damaged. But if I cannot will this in my own case,
> how can I consistently deny to others the right to life that I claim for

myself? I would break the so-called Golden Rule, unless I denied that a mother had in general a right to an abortion.

1(b).

Everybody has certain rights over his or her body. To establish such rights we need merely show that it cannot be shown that anyone else has a right to interfere with the implementation of our own desires about our bodies. It follows that at the stage when the embryo is essentially part of the mother's body, the mother has the right to make her own uncoerced decision on whether she will have an abortion or not. Since she has her moral right, she ought also to have a legal right.

2(a).

A physician should decide whether to tell a patient who is gravely ill or dying about his or her condition by reckoning on the consequences in that particular case to that particular patient of giving or withholding that specific information. If the patient's health and happiness will be increased by telling the truth, then the truth should be told; but if not, not so.

2(b).

To treat an agent with moral respect is to look to his dignity and not his happiness. To deprive a man of the truth about his disease or his death is to deprive him of dignity. More particularly every man can only respect himself if he faces up to the fact of his own death. Hence to deprive patients of the truth about themselves is to do them a wrong and a wrong that insults their status as human beings.

3(a).

Justice demands that every citizen should have so far as is possible an equal chance to develop his talents and his other potentialities. But good health is a prerequisite for such development. Therefore every citizen should have an equal right to access to the means of good health, so far as it is available. Therefore justice requires a free national health service, financed out of taxation, with no private sector of medical practice.

3(b).

Everybody has a right to incur only such obligations as he chooses, to be free to make such contracts as he wishes. Every doctor must therefore be free to accept patients or not and to practice on what terms he chooses. If others then do not wish to deal with him, that is their free choice. Freedom of contract requires medicine to be a matter of private practice.[5]

The first argument pits our moral intuitions about the generalizability of moral judgments against our respect for bodily integrity. The second opposes health, and perhaps even life, to honesty. The third reveals social welfare once again in conflict with individual freedom. I agree with MacIntyre that such dilemmas hold the makings of tragedy.

There is no rational method of resolving these disputes, MacIntyre argues, because those who accept the premises of rival arguments share no common moral ground. And this, presumably, is because we have "no rationally defensible concept of man's true end or of an essential human nature." Instead, all we have in our moral arsenal is a "collection of fragments"—moral principles of a variety of sorts available for assertion from a variety of moral points of view. I believe this characterization of our moral plight, on which characterization MacIntyre's argument essentially depends, fails to do justice to what we know about moral reasoning. In order to challenge his gloomy conclusions about what philosophy can say to the moral problems in medical practice, I must therefore offer a different perspective on that plight.

The moral principles that we espouse are indeed in conflict. One must sometimes lie to keep a promise, inflict pain to save a life, or sacrifice efficiency to protect autonomy. In some cases of such conflict, no real dilemma is involved. When we stopped to save the drowning child, we were not in conflict, even though a promised appointment would therefore not be kept. Yet we retain our belief that it is good to keep promises. But sometimes the conflict does involve dilemma, and the cases drawn from medicine are paradigmatic of this sort. In such cases, principles of value can conflict so as to cause substantial distress. One does not know which of the competing principles to honor; instead, one suffers the anxiety of moral uncertainty. Can we reasonably blame our lack of a global moral outlook for our distress? Is it true that we are resourceless, that the proponents of rival moral arguments share no common moral ground?

The moral principles that we honor are not simply a random collection of ancient ethical artifacts. On the contrary, they are the expression of values that we accept—which is to say, descriptions of goods that we want. Each moral theory that has any plausibility depends for its hearing on the fact that it captures the essence of at least some part of what we take to have moral significance: In the case of utilitarianism it is our commitment to beneficence that underlies the theory; in the case of libertarianism it is our respect for personal autonomy that informs the moral view; in the case of a Kantian outlook our concerns for the moral force of reason and for the integrity of our relationships with other people are central ingredients. There are many goods that we want, among them respect for bodily integrity, honesty, individual freedom, and health. Nagel, similarly, speaks of "economic, political and personal liberty, equality, equity, privacy, procedural fairness, intellectual and aesthetic development, community, general utility, desert," and others.[6] The principles corresponding to these various goods survive because these are values that we do hold, and the importance we attach to each principle reflects the centrality of the corresponding value.

These principles, it is important to recall, pertain to actions; moral judgment, after all, is primarily judgment about how people ought to act. But man as a moral agent faces a morally recalcitrant world. I do not refer to the behavior of others. I refer, rather, to the fact that in many ways that matter, we simply cannot have what we want. There is nothing contradictory about the concept of a world in which relief of suffering and the prolongation of life are never in conflict. There is nothing in logic to preclude a world in which patients are never at risk of being injured by the truth. Indeed, there is no conceptual flaw in a world of perfect health. But these are not our world. Instead, man as a moral agent often faces life like the hungry dieter confronted with a hot fudge sundae. He can imagine a world in which his hunger would be satisfied with a single bite; he can contemplate a world in which such delicacies are not fattening. But in this world his desires are in conflict. Ambivalence is his state; dilemma, his burden; regret, his likely companion. Yet there is nothing inappropriate in wanting to be fed but not fat. He is thwarted by the empirical world, not by any incoherence in his desires.

What, then, of the physician who respects life and respects a pregnant woman's bodily integrity, who is convinced by argument (1a) that he ought not to perform a requested abortion and is convinced by argument (1b) that he ought to perform it? Must he flit, like the characters in Tom Stoppard's philosophical play *Jumpers*,[7] from stance to stance, unable to find any basis for landing on either side of the issue? Like our hungry dieter, he will be ambivalent, and he will recognize in the conflict he faces the moral recalcitrance of the real world. But he is not necessarily resourceless, any more than the hungry dieter is resourceless. For the dieter can acknowledge that delicious food is good and fattening food is bad, can recognize that the object of his judgment bears many attributes, including those of being delicious and being fattening, and can then adopt a broader perspective in his quest for decision. He can reflect, for example, that the aspirations that inform what he presently sees as his rational life plan would be advanced more substantially by weight reduction than by immediate gastronomic gratification and thus may abstain—with regret at what he thereby misses conjoined with satisfaction at what he thereby gains. Or he may decide that his deprivation has been so sustained and his progress so substantial that the incorporation of inspiring ingestible incentives is deserved and prudent. In either case, he gets off dead center by relating the conflicting arguments to a broader prudential context in terms of which he can override one in favor of the other. He takes into account both of the conflicting arguments and reconciles the conflict by judging them against an overriding purpose—not, to be sure, an overriding purpose that informs all human actions; merely a purpose that is overriding with respect to the two alternative actions under consideration. But that is overriding enough.

Can the troubled physician not do the same, resolving his dilemma in terms of a broader *moral* perspective that enables him to choose between two troubling alternatives? That he can is precisely what MacIntyre denies. Recall his explicit assertion that "those who accept the premises of rival arguments share no common moral ground." Yet the rivals in question may well be—indeed, often are—just two different facets of the moral reasoning of one individual faced with a choice. Why is there no common moral ground? Presumably because the conflicting principles are unrelated fragments from the past, cut adrift from the cohesive foundation that can be provided only by a sense of man's true end or essential nature.

I believe a different description of our moral circumstances is needed here. The agent faced with moral dilemma who is thus in internal moral conflict and the separate moral adversaries, too, may find no common ground in the premises of the moral arguments they accept. But MacIntyre has offered us no argument that shows they cannot find common moral ground by expanding the scope of their deliberations. Consider a case in point. A child in the advanced stages of Hurler's disease falls ill with a life-threatening infection. His disease is a grotesque, degenerative, terminal illness. His infection is readily treatable. Should the physician cure the infection, thus saving the child's life for a brief period of continued degradation, frustration, and suffering? Opinion A argues for treatment, citing the invariant value and sanctity of life and the physician's consequent obligation always to strive to preserve it. Opinion B argues against treatment, citing the value of kindness, of welcoming the benevolent intervention of natural events in a chilling human tragedy. Have they truly no common moral ground?

Let us press B and ask why he opposes medical intervention to thwart the infection. It is plausible to assume that he will cite such factors as the pain suffered by the patient and his family, the utter hopelessness of Hurler's disease, the draining costs, psychic as well as monetary, of keeping the patient alive, and all the rest. Under further questioning he may allow that these outcomes are undesirable because they constitute or cause agonizing experiences for all concerned, including the patient. Allowing the patient's life to end, on the other hand, will minimize such experience. Now let us press A and ask him why he holds life to be always worth preserving. There are many answers he might give, foreshadowed in the debate among the four physicians in chapter 4. He might argue that where there is life, there is hope, suggesting that a cure for the disease may be announced at any moment. He might argue that medical research always stands to gain from considering the seriously ill. The longer the patient survives, the more data are available. He may assert that life simply is of intrinsic and overriding worth and thus should be preserved no matter what. Each of these three responses, of course, reflects a significantly different moral basis for the view that life has value. Finally, he may observe that life has value because it is a prerequisite for the experiences that alone have intrinsic value.

I readily admit that the conversation might not go like that. But assume that it does. Then, if A can be convinced that there is no significant prospect of the patient's having valuable future experiences or contributing to valuable future experiences of others, whatever such experiences are taken to be, A may relinquish the view that *this* patient's life is valuable at this time, holding now to the view that life for the most part, precisely because it is the precondition of the experiences that constitute the basis of value, is of overriding importance. A and B may then agree.

Again, I do not argue that the story *must* follow this course. There may instead be an intractable clash of viewpoints. I argue only that the story *might* follow this course. And if it does, then we have an instance wherein moral conflict is resolved precisely because the adversaries have come to see that there is, or have come to adopt, a common moral ground after all, despite their having begun with opposing views derived from ostensibly irreconcilable moral positions.

It is important to be clear about how this resolution has proceeded. The conflict has not been dispelled in any *ad hoc* way. Rather, three systematic steps have led to a mutually acknowledged general principle. First, the disputants examined the reasons and presuppositions that supported their rival positions. Secondly, they identified in those presuppositions the common moral ground that experiences alone have intrinsic value. Thirdly, they abstracted from that common moral ground to a principle that resolves the present case: Life is valuable only because of, and therefore only in the presence of, valuable experience or the possibility of valuable experience. This principle is generalizable, however, to other cases and constitutes a more basic level of moral judgment for both disputants than their original rival premises.

Of course, nothing in this example shows the principle to be incontrovertible. It is not self-certifying, nor has it been shown to be the conclusion of a valid argument with incontrovertible premises. Thus, even if we are inclined to accept the principle, we can maintain a residual uncertainty about whether action based on it is right from the perspective of eternity, as the philosophers like to say. If MacIntyre's point is simply that such certification is unavailable, I quite agree. But that, of course, has nothing whatever to do with the ability of philosophy to help find common moral ground between disputants where it does exist or to help fashion it where it can exist. And if that common moral ground lies within morally acceptable borders, some progress will indeed have then been made. That is, if that common moral ground satisfies the conditions of respect for persons—for some reasonable mix of their rights and their interests—then some relief from moral dilemma may follow.

Or is this overly optimistic? Perhaps I have based the point on a case of my own invention and inferred too much from the result. The challenge of MacIntyre's moral skepticism would be more effectively met if the response were based on the very dilemmas that he has used to illustrate the hopelessness of the quest for moral solutions.

8

Resolving Moral Conflict: The Response

To CONSIDER MacIntyre's three examples of moral conflict, imagine a dialogue about each of them. The speakers are two physicians, Drs. Ernest Healer and Patience Care, joined by Minerva, the ancient goddess of the liberal arts, flown in for the occasion. The discussion begins with the second conflict, about revealing the truth to a dying patient.

C: My position is given in 2(a). The truth can sometimes be ruinous to a patient we are trying to help. There is no justification for that. Depending on a patient's condition, the truth can be brutal, damaging, and misleading. We have to decide on the basis of what is best for the patient.

H: And my position is given in 2(b). We have no right to withhold the truth from any patient; to do so is an act of arrogant disrespect. In regard to dying patients, a conspiracy of secrecy is particularly loathsome; it prevents them from coming to terms honestly with the final stage of life.

M: You two are disagreeing pretty sharply over this issue. I wonder if there is any prospect for diminishing the disagreement. I'd like to probe your positions a bit more deeply, to see if there is any possibility of accommodation.

C: That's fine. But I don't have much sympathy for his rigid absolutism.

H: Nor I for her willingness to manipulate what other people can know about themselves according to what she thinks is good for them. But go ahead.

M: All right. Dr. Healer, do you believe, as Kant did, that it is always wrong to tell a lie? Or do you think it is sometimes justified? I have in mind cases where a lot is at stake. I'm sure you know the sorts of cases that make the point. A homicidal maniac, escaped from custody, has vowed to kill the judge who sentenced him. The judge is hiding to the left; the police are hiding to the right, set to recapture the killer. He stops in front of you and asks which way the judge went. And he trusts you. Do you tell him the truth or lie?

H: That's no problem. I'm not the rigid absolutist I'm accused of being. I'd lie in that case; I'm sure most people would. But, you see, I'm not lying to a patient then. I'm not lying to someone I have special obligations toward. I don't owe him anything. I have a duty to society that requires the lie. That has nothing to do with a dying patient. And it has nothing to do with the medical profession, to which I also have an obligation—to help maintain a climate of trust between patients and the profession.

C: It's just silly to think that confidence in the medical profession is going to crumble if a patient is actually benefited once in a while from a bit of judicious deception.

M: Now, let's not jump ahead too fast. So far we've agreed that some conditions justify deception. We agree to at least that little bit, don't we?

H: We do.

C: But we don't agree about what the conditions are.

M: Yes, that is true. But let's see what principle lies behind the bit of agreement we do have. Dr. Healer, you don't think the situation I described is a good analogy to the kinds of cases this dispute is about. But let's stay with that situation a little longer. Do you agree that in general lying is wrong, that unless there is some special justification for a lie, one ought to tell the truth?

H: Of course. I believe in honesty as a fundamental value. She's the one who's ready to play fast and loose with it.

M: Let's leave out the insults and try to understand each other's views. Now, you agree that honesty is a fundamental value. Yet you also agree that sometimes a lie can be justified. Why? What can justify the lie in those cases where you agree that it can be told?

H: You said it yourself before. Where there is a lot at stake. Where the truth could cost an innocent life, like the life of your judge.

M: But now there seems to be a problem about the medical situations. At least with cases where a life may hang in the balance. Remember Mr. Angstimmer in chapter 3? We had to keep him quiet to help him recover from his heart attack. If we told him what we knew about his neurological results, we would fuel irrational fears and maybe kill him. So there was a lot at stake. Don't you agree that deception was right in that situation?

C: Of course. That's just the kind of case.

H: No, not at all. I mean, yes, the deception then was right. But it was to save his life, not to hide the truth that he was dying. And it was just a delay. To keep him alive. If he recovers, comes out of intensive care, then we tell him when he is stable, and we can help him handle the information. I never said that we have to go in with bad news like marines at a beachhead.

M: But what principle justifies the way we manage the information? Is it something we do out of beneficence?

H: Yes, beneficence. But also a respect for his autonomy. If he's dead, there's no autonomy, there's nothing to respect.

M: So we withhold the truth from him for his own good?

H: In that case, yes.

M: You seem to have come a long way from your statement that to deprive patients of the truth about themselves is to do them a wrong, to deprive them of dignity.

H: Perhaps I have to qualify it a bit, but not much. It is usually a wrong. I only agreed that in a few cases—where life is at stake—then it might be a right.

M: But it is not always a wrong, not absolutely?

H: No.

M: Then your view does turn out to be less rigid than it seemed. Perhaps Dr. Care's view is not quite what it appears either.

C: What do you mean?

M: You say that patients with grave or terminal illness should be told the truth or not depending on the physician's judgment about what will increase the patient's health and happiness. Is that right?

C: Yes. And that is why a case with life at stake is so easy. Of course, we should lie to save a life; that is necessary to increase health and happiness.

M: If you had a grave illness, would you want to know about it?

C: Yes, I would. But not if the knowledge would kill me sooner. But some people would not want to know at all.

M: How do you tell that? How can you decide what amount of truth will be best for a patient's health and happiness?

C: Well, it can be hard, I admit. Usually the patients let you know. If they really want the truth, they ask, they press for it. Sometimes they just know. Nothing has been said explicitly. But they know, and they don't want it out in the open. They aren't able to handle it, or they are protecting the family. Something like that. It takes getting to know them, and treading very lightly at first, until you have a sense of how much they can handle.

H: That's what I object to. Most physicians hardly know their patients anymore, at least in any deep way. It's such a superficial judgment. You can't even be sure how someone you've known for years is going to react to shocking news. It's just a pretension to think we can decide wisely what a patient can handle. All this talk about treading lightly is just a smoke screen to hide the fact that there is no real basis for predicting what the effect will be of learning that one is dying or gravely ill.

M: Hold on a minute. I don't want to get into a debate about how well you can tell what a patient can handle because I don't understand the question. What do you mean when you speak of handling the information? What counts as handling it or as failing to handle it?

C: It means not being made worse. You gave an example. The man in the cardiac ICU—if he got so upset at the information that he went into arrest, I would say that he did not handle the information.

M: But we've all agreed about that case. What about the patient who does not have any dramatic physical deterioration on hearing the grim news but who gets very upset—weepy, depressed, discouraged?

C: Yes, that would be something to avoid.

M: By withholding the truth?

C: Yes.

M: But why? Why is that something to avoid?

C: Because it lessens health and happiness. The patient is worse off.

M: All right. Now let's take a short detour. If your friend has written some dreadful poetry and asks you, as a friend, to give an honest opinion of the poetry, what do you do?

C: You have to say that maybe poetry isn't the best mode of expression for that person. You don't have to say it is dreadful. But you can't say it is very good. I'm assuming your friend really wants to know. Maybe to avoid the embarrassment of showing it to others; maybe that's the reason for asking a friend who can be trusted to tell the truth.

M: And if your friend is sensitive and will become discouraged if you are truthful? And you know it?

C: Still, you have to get the idea across that it isn't good. You can try to put it gently.

M: And if you do that—put it gently—but the friend still gets upset, weeps for a while, gets discouraged, and gives up writing poetry, have you done the right thing?

C: I would have to say yes. Maybe it is good that the poetry stops if the reality is that it is dreadful. You've upset the friend for a while, but it can pass.

M: And you have done a good thing because you have helped the friend come to terms with reality?

C: Yes.

M: Even though the friend is upset at first?

C: Yes. Because maybe the friend wanted to be a poet. But it wouldn't have been possible anyway. Sooner or later that ambition would be thwarted.

M: And you would say that the friend was able to handle the bad news? With the weeping and depression and discouragement?

C: I see what you're after now. I have to say yes and no. The friend didn't take it well at first. But after that it was handled. Unless—we don't know enough about the case—unless the friend doesn't recover from the depression.

M: And even then is it your fault? Or were you right to tell the truth, to give the friend the opportunity to handle the truth well or badly?

C: I guess it would be right even then. Unless you knew that the friend couldn't take it. Then maybe I would not be honest. If I knew the friend was so fragile as to be unable to recover from the truth.

M: Do you have any friends like that? Who are so fragile that you are sure they could not take the truth?

C: Not that I'm sure of. I know some doubtful cases, that's for sure. Some people I consider pretty fragile. But not enough to convince me in advance that it would be a mistake to give them an honest reaction. But I would go very indirectly with some of them.

M: So now—and I'm sure you've expected this by now—tell me how it is different with a patient. And I mean a patient who is dying or gravely ill, someone who probably wants to be well, just as your friend may want to be a good poet. But it isn't to be. And the truth may cause depression. But of course, it is depressing truth. How is this case different? You see, you didn't say that you would be honest or not with the friend depending on your assessment of what would produce the most happiness.

C: Because you can't be a friend like that—constantly calculating the consequences of what you say. There has to be more trust, more honesty, or you don't really have a friendship. But you have a special obligation to do what is best for your patients. You have to calculate the consequences there.

M: And what counts as good consequences? If your patient becomes hysterical, then despondent, then gradually accepts the situation and sets his affairs in order, is that a good or a bad outcome? Has the patient handled the truth well enough or not?

H: There's no possible answer to that. She can't say. It isn't up to anyone else to judge that as good or bad. The person faces the illness, the death, one way or another. Maybe with acceptance, and maybe with unrelenting rage. But it is his own way, and nobody has a right to deny him that.

M: Do you agree with that?

C: Not quite. But I do see the force of it. I don't feel very comfortable now with my ability to say what a good outcome is. I see that a lot of emotional upheaval might take place, without that being a reason to deceive the patient. But still, I think there are outcomes so bad that they justify deception. Like killing the patient with the news.

H: I've already agreed to that.

C: But short of that, it is hard to say. A patient might get despondent and commit suicide.

H: What's wrong with that if it's the patient's decision?

M: That's a related topic, of course—the question of the right to take one's own life. But we do have two other conflicts to consider, so I'd rather not face that one just now. Let's see if we can sum up where we are in respect to telling the truth. Do you see your positions as changed now, either of you?

H: Well, somewhat. I see that sometimes the price for telling the truth is higher than I'd be willing to pay. When there is a strong case that it would have a permanently damaging effect on the patient. So I can't make the principle absolute. But I'm still committed to honesty in most cases. I do agree that the presentation of the information requires some sensitivity.

C: Yes, I've changed my views a bit, too. I don't have as much confidence as I did in my sense of what deception is aimed at preventing. So I would be more inclined to tell the truth. I do see the point about being able to face one's own end well or badly, in one's own way. But I would still be more inclined than Dr. Healer to mask the truth. The reality is sometimes so tragic that I am not inclined to make people stare it in the face if I think they will just come apart. I'm not as hostile to some comforting self-deception, and I'm even willing to be an accomplice. But I think I will be less likely now to see a case as justifying that kind of handling. So I've moved a little closer to his position.

M: So there is still some area of disagreement. You'd draw the lines in different places. But that area of disagreement has shrunk a little. You both see the value of truthfulness as required for respecting the patient's dignity and right to face tragedy well or badly in his own way. And you both agree that sometimes it is justified to override that value to avoid very likely very bad consequences. Is that right?

H: Yes.

C: That's right.

M: And where you disagree concerns how certain or how bad the consequences have to be to justify deception?

C: And, to some extent, what counts as a bad outcome.

H: Yes, since I think it is sometimes an acceptable outcome for a patient to end his life. I even think that part of the case for honesty is to allow that choice.

M: So we have made some progress, and I think we can go on to another conflict. Let's consider the argument about private practice and a national health service.

C: I'm for a national health service. I gave my reasons in 3(b).

H: And I believe in freedom. My view is 3(a).

M: I suspect these views aren't isolated from your more general political outlooks. Is that right?

C: It sure is. I think he's a reactionary of the worst sort. His ideal society is the Wild West or at least the nineteenth century. Rugged individualism, every man for himself, face up to your responsibilities, and all of that. And he thinks I'm a soppy, bleeding-heart do-gooder.

H: She is.

C: You see?

M: I see, at least, that we have a serious issue to deal with here. You say—and I'm sure it's true—that good health is a prerequisite to the development of one's talents and potentialities. Is it the only prerequisite?

C: I suppose not. Of course, the basic necessities have to be available: food, shelter, clothing. No one should have to go without those either.

M: And so they should also be provided by a free national service—a national food, shelter, and clothing service?

C: For those who need it, yes. That's what we do; we provide the basic necessities through social welfare programs to those who can't survive otherwise. I wouldn't want to be part of a society so inhumane as to abandon people who are destitute, no matter what the reasons for their condition.

M: Now I am a bit puzzled. A moment ago you were talking about the development of talents; now you are talking about survival. It takes a lot more to enable someone to develop talents than just to ensure survival.

C: Well, of course, it does. But you have to start with survival. That's the minimum. You can't just let people starve or die of exposure. And you have to treat them when their lives are threatened by illness and injury. And then you go beyond that, so that they can develop. That's why we have education; it is free, and it is for everyone of school age, not just for those who can afford it.

H: But our economy is at the point of collapse from social programs already. Add a national health service, and we'll fall apart economically. Besides, people should pay their own way. We don't give free food, shelter, or clothing to most people. Why should we give free health service to everyone? And who is supposed to pay for it all?

M: That's a lot of questions all at once. Let's try to keep the focus sharp. We're talking about the development of talents and what that takes. And we see that a system of free public education helps meet that need. But is it enough? I have in mind a young man who wants to be a drama critic and is very poor. Should the government pay for his theater tickets? What of his friend who wants to be a good skier—not as a profession—it is just a talent he wants to develop? Should the government pay for his trip to the mountains?

C: Of course not. I haven't said that everything anyone wants should be free.

M: But you do see that in these cases they need expensive things to develop these potentials?

C: Well, yes. But they have to make some sacrifice themselves. They can get jobs, take loans, maybe work part time to pay for the extra costs.

M: And if there are no jobs or if they can't find work?

C: Then they may not be able to get what they want. But those are not necessities—theater tickets and ski trips. They are luxuries they can live quite well without.

M: Then it sounds as if we are moving back in the direction of survival's being the issue. Because if these things, which are necessary to the development of the talents in question, are luxuries, then maybe all the things that go beyond survival are luxuries. Or if not, how do you separate what the state should provide from what goes beyond that level?

C: That is a problem. But let me see if I can say something reasonable about it. The state should provide people with those things that *everyone* needs, like food and shelter, that they can't provide for themselves.

H: And open heart surgery? Not everyone needs that.

C: But everyone needs health care. That's what should be provided, depending on what the particular needs are.

M: And everyone needs some goods beyond the level of survival in order to develop talents. Like education. So that should be provided, depending on the particular needs. Is that right?

C: Yes, that's right.

M: Like, in the cases we just considered, tickets and trips?

C: No. I guess I just haven't got it clear enough yet. But I'm just not willing to turn my back on people who need medical help.

M: I wonder if perhaps you haven't thought enough about what your reason for that is. At first it was in terms of developing talents. But that led to some confusion. That doesn't show your conclusion is wrong. Maybe you just need a better argument for it.

C: I'd love one. What do you have to offer?

M: I'm afraid I'll have to disappoint you here. You have to do your own work! I'll just suggest that you think harder about why you think health care should be provided free to everyone when it doesn't really seem to be based on the development of talents. What are the basic reasons?

C: It starts with a respect for people. They are all of value, as individuals. So their needs are important. Some of them can get along fine on their own, but some are disadvantaged. It often isn't their fault; it is just the circumstances they are in. So they need extra help, extra support. Some of us are very lucky. We have good jobs, good educations, often because we had the advantage of a good background. How can we justify living so well and having more than others? We have to make up for the advantages in some way, by being concerned with the disadvantaged people. It's as Rawls says. We should be judged by how we treat the least well-off. And we should justify our advantages in terms of helping those who are at the bottom of society. It is a question of justice. Those who have had the chance to develop their talents should help make it possible for others. And we do that partly through the government, by providing what people need.

M: That they can't afford on their own?

C: Right.

M: Then how does that show that there should be a free national health service, rather than a system of health care that is available free just to those who cannot afford their own health care insurance?

C: Well, I guess it doesn't show that. It depends, I guess, on whether you see health care as being as important as education. We let people have private schools if they want it. But we provide free public education to everyone, rich or poor alike. I think health care is as important.

M: But can it be just a question of importance? Certainly food is even more important than education. But we don't provide food to everyone. We just provide it to the poor who would starve otherwise. So why shouldn't we just provide health care to those who would otherwise be unable to get it?

C: I don't know. Maybe that would work. I'm just not sure at this point. But I know that I just can't accept the idea that private practice is enough to provide fair access to medical care for everyone. Private practice means that people who can't pay can be denied medical care completely. He may not care about that, but I do.

H: That is a complete distortion! Of course, I care about medical care for anyone who needs it. But that doesn't mean that I can disregard the rights of doctors. I think anyone who has any sense, who can afford it, will have a good health insurance policy. Usually it will be provided by an employer. So all those people are covered—with their families. That's most people right there. Some people are wealthy and would rather insure themselves. That's fine. That leaves the poor people. Now there's no excuse for saying that just because someone is in private practice, he doesn't care about the poor. In my group we always have a collection of reduced-fee and no-fee patients. That's maybe ten or twelve percent of our time. And we do this because we do care about medical care for poor people. But nobody has a right to come along and tell us we have to. That would be a violation of our rights as individuals in a free society. I'm against compulsion, not compassion.

C: But that just misses the point completely. It isn't enough that some poor people are fortunate enough to come across this great compassion. What about the ones who aren't near practices like that? Don't they have a right to treatment, too? Your compassion doesn't do a thing for the old lady in the ghetto who is too sick to come out to your fancy clinic.

H: You can't expect the medical profession to solve the problems of society. The poor are poor because they don't work. Maybe that's because there are no jobs for them. It doesn't matter. It is an economic problem, not a medical one. If the government worried less about trying to make everyone happy and healthy and stuck to its proper business of protection of the rights of individuals, there would be a healthier economy and fewer poor patients to worry about. In the meantime, I do my best to live up to my contracts with my patients, and other good doctors do the same. We can't solve everyone's problems.

M: I'm glad you've raised the question of contracts again because I've been wondering about that since you first stated your position.

H: What question? I believe in freedom of contract, but I didn't raise any question about it.

M: But you did indeed, at least in my mind. You believe in a minimal role for government; is that right?

H: Yes. Nozick has the right idea, not Rawls.

M: And you also take contracts very seriously?

H: Of course. Contracts create rights. So my patients have a right to my services, but only when I accept them as patients.

M: Do they actually sign written contracts that spell out the rights and responsibilities that each of you has?

H: No, of course not. That's hardly possible—I mean, to spell it all out completely. But there are understandings and expectations. If you like, it could be considered an implicit contract.

M: Yes, I understand. And even though the contract is implicit, you still take it seriously?

H: Of course.

M: Are the only contracts you have with your patients? Or are there others also?

H: Many others. With the company that owns our building. With our staff. Suppliers. Insurance companies. Contractual understandings and individual rights are the fabric of society.

M: And what about your family? Do you have a family?

H: Yes.

M: And do you have contracts with your wife and children?

H: Yes, in a way. Not formal contracts, of course. But there is a relationship there, and it gives rise to expectations and understandings about what each one owes the other. So it is a sort of tacit contract, too.

M: Now who gave you your license to practice medicine? Was it a group of patients?

H: No, it comes from the state.

M: And could you practice medicine without it?

H: Not legally.

M: So it is a benefit for you to have it?

H: Yes. A benefit I earned.

M: And does it carry certain responsibilities along with it? A sort of contract between you and the state?

H: In a way. I have to practice according to the law.

M: And if the law required that you devote a certain percentage of your time to treating the poor?

H: It doesn't. And that would be bad law.

M: Still, there could be such a law. And everyone is free not to become a doctor. So if there were such a law—or if there had been—you would not have been forced to accept the conditions. But they would have been the price you would have had to pay to receive the license. A part of the contract?

H: Yes. But I might have chosen to go into carpentry instead.

M: Now, what about your medical education. Wasn't that a benefit of a very great sort?

H: Of course it was.

M: And don't you owe society something in return?

H: What I owe is being the best physician I can. As far as the cost is concerned, I paid my own way. Borrowed tens of thousands, and it took years to pay it all back. That was a contract, and I met my side of the bargain.

M: So in the end you had paid for your own medical education?

H: Yes.

M: And does that mean that you paid the tuition, or did you also reimburse the school for your share of the initial capital investment in building it?

H: The tuition. And all the other expenses. But medical students aren't expected to cover capitalization costs.

M: Who does?

H: It depends on the age of the school. A lot of it was built with federal grants.

M: The public, in other words?

H: I suppose so.

M: And what about your medical knowledge? The information you have about your medical specialty. Isn't that a valuable asset in your profession?

H: Essential. Why? What are you driving at?

M: You'll see soon enough. Do you, along with the other physicians, pay for the costs of medical research—for the development of the knowledge that you learned in medical school and since?

H: No, we don't pay for that directly. Medical research is financed separately for the most part. In practice, we use the results as well as we can. If the research stopped, the practice of medicine would go on. But the quality would stop improving.

M: But you couldn't go on without the knowledge that was developed in the past.

H: No, we couldn't.

M: And who paid for that?

H: A lot of people. Over the generations. It builds up over time. Some of it is done by individuals—but not so much anymore. Some of it was supported by drug companies. Or done in universities. Most of it is supported by public funds. It all adds up; it is a part of our common scientific heritage.

M: Would it be fair to say that it belongs to society as a whole?

H: I don't see why not.

M: And that in agreeing to convey it to you—especially by allocating to you one of those extremely rare medical school seats—society made available to you a substantial benefit, largely supported by public funds, without which you could not be a physician at all?

H: I suppose so.

M: Then is it entirely implausible to believe that you have certain obligations in return? That there is an implicit contract between you and the larger society that has made it possible for you to enjoy the benefits of being a physician? And that a part of that obligation is to care for those who cannot afford care?

H: I won't say that it is entirely implausible. But that is a pretty tenuous argument—and a wrong one, I think—when you get to the details of the obligations. I think my obligations are to my profession and to my patients.

M: But you agree at least that there are obligations that go along with the benefits of a medical education and a medical license?

H: Yes.

M: And that the contract that exists between the doctor and the society is an implicit one, not an explicit one?

H: Right.

M: And that there is some room for disagreement about just what is involved in that implicit agreement?

H: Yes, I suppose there is room for disagreement. It would depend on a lot of broad issues about the relationship between the individual and his society.

C: I think the trouble here is that there is no explicit agreement, nothing to make him see what his obligations really are. It should be made clear. A license to practice medicine is a great privilege. It should be considered a public trust. Considering the extent of public investment over the years that is relied on in training any one physician, and considering the importance to the population of having a good and just system of health care, I think it would even make sense to consider medicine a public utility and to regulate it accordingly. It is just as important as communications or power.

H: You're advocating an obsolete notion. Even the government is recognizing the dangers of regulation and is deregulating communications and other industries. Not fast enough, but very noticeably. But even a regulated industry is better than a socialized one. A public utility is not the same as a nationalized service.

M: Now, before we go too far afield, I want to get back to your original argument. Let's put aside, for the moment, the question of a national health service. And let's set aside the question of regulating health care as a public utility. Do you agree, at least, that the physician has obligations to society in recognition of the substantial social investment that enabled him to become a physician?

H: Yes, I've agreed to that.

M: And these obligations, whatever they are, place some limits on what the physician may do? Limits that, if we stay with the contract metaphor, are part of the terms of the implicit contract between the physician and his society?

H: Yes.

M: But you have said that every doctor must be free to practice on what terms he chooses. That sounds like a more unrestrained kind of freedom to practice than you really believe in.

H: I see that I wasn't clear enough or careful enough. You know, it's easy to forget that philosophy demands being careful just as much as medicine does. So I'd have to put it a little differently, I suppose.

M: How?

H: That doctors must be free to practice as they choose, within the limits of law and of their obligations.

M: And those obligations could include some responsibility to make social contributions, to care for needy patients?

H: That would have to be shown.

M: But it is not impossible?

H: I don't see how to show it is impossible.

M: Now I think we've made some progress here. If I've followed our discussion correctly, you've both modified your positions somewhat. Dr. Care, you're no longer convinced that the case for a national health service rests on a just concern for the opportunities people have to develop their talents. You've maintained your commitment to meeting the health care needs of the disadvantaged, but you're no longer sure that a national health service, supported by taxation, is the only acceptable way to do it. Is that a fair description?

C: Yes, I think that's fair.

M: And you, Dr. Healer, are still firmly committed to private practice. But you do have a concern with the health care needs of the poor. And you do recognize that physicians cannot justly have complete freedom, but only freedom within the limits of the implicit contract they have with the larger society that has trained them and that legitimizes their position as physicians.

C: A very privileged position.

H: Yes, that's a fair description of my view. But I'm not apologetic about the privilege, nor do I feel the least bit guilty about it, as I suspect Dr. Care does. We earn it through skill, hard work, long hours, high risks, and doing good for others.

M: Now it's clear, I think, that your views are still fairly far apart. And it's equally clear that each of you can find a lot of supporters; there's nothing particularly idiosyncratic about either of your positions. But you're both members of the same community, and only one policy can be in effect. So what do you propose to do? What can you do?

H: I can keep advocating my views and living by them.

C: And I can try to get people to see that we are not doing enough.

M: And in the meantime?

H: It's a matter of politics. Of who has the votes.

C: But it's also a matter of right, of fighting for a just society no matter what the votes are like.

M: But people disagree about what justice is and what it requires. Do you see people who won't agree with you as evil?

H: Not evil, no. I see some of them as misguided, though.

C: Yet you have modified your own views somewhat already. So perhaps you were a bit misguided yourself.

H: Yes. But my basic outlook is the same. It's just that I understand a bit better what my beliefs are, and I see more clearly some of the complications in getting them right.

M: And do you see the views of the other side any differently?

H: Somewhat. At least she's backed off nationalization a bit, and it's more a question now of social obligations.

M: And you see that as closer to your own views.

H: Closer, but still quite different.

M: Do you agree?

C: I do, yes. He's not been quite as rigid as his argument at first. So maybe I could persuade him to accept some sort of structure that would meet the needs of everyone.

M: At least I think you both can see that we're dealing with an exceedingly complex matter here, and it is unlikely that you would ever reach complete agreement. But each of you has been able to see weaknesses in your own argument. And if we had the time, I'm sure you would each come to see some strengths in the other argument—at least in the values that give rise to it. So there should be some basis for carrying the discussion forward. Even if you reach a compromise solution at the level of policy, it will have to reflect the diversity of opinions that are politically prominent, so few people will likely be completely happy with it. It will likely be an unstable solution. But it might be one that you both can live with.

C: I think, anyway, we have a basis for continuing the discussion. I see it as the question of what the physician's obligations to society are.

H: Yes, that's the question. So we have what I think the diplomats call a framework for discussion. That means we now agree on what we disagree about!

M: Good. Then, lest our readers abandon us in despair, we'd best get on to the last set of arguments, the ones about abortion. I've deliberately left this one to last because it may be the most difficult of the three. So let's begin with a review of your positions.

H: My position is given in argument 1(a); I'm essentially a Kantian with respect to matters of morality. I cannot will for another what I cannot will for myself, so I can only be an opponent of abortion and a defender of the right to life for all.

C: And my position is given in 1(b). The right of autonomy over one's own body gives every woman the right not to be pregnant if she does not want to be, even if that means having an abortion.

M: I wonder if I understand your initial positions well enough. I'd like to try to get them somewhat clearer.

H: Sure.

C: Go ahead.

M: All right. Now let's start with the question of bodily integrity. Dr. Care, if I understand you correctly, your argument in support of a right to abortion is based on a belief about bodily integrity, about our right to exercise autonomy in regard to what happens to our bodies. Is that right?

C: Yes, that's it.

M: But there is something about your argument that I find troublesome. Let me try to get at it by a somewhat indirect route. Are you in favor of making prostitution legal?

C: Prostitution? I don't know. What has that to do with the matter?

M: Just this, that if people have a right to do as they wish with their own bodies, then women should have the right to be prostitutes if they choose, shouldn't they?

C: I suppose that's so. Anyway, I see your reasoning. So let's say yes, I would have to allow prostitution to be legal. But I might still want to argue that it isn't a very healthy thing. You know, like smoking. I don't say that it should be against the law, but it is a stupid, even a tragic kind of behavior.

M: All right. Now, do you write prescriptions for your patients?

C: Of course. When they need them. Why?

M: Only that the whole system of prescription writing is based on the idea that certain drugs should be regulated. If all drugs were available over the counter, you could just tell your patients what to take, and they could go get whatever they wanted from the pharmacy. Would you favor that?

C: No, no. Patients can't just handle their own medication. They'd kill themselves, some of them. They don't know enough about drugs. As it is, it's often a problem to get them to handle drugs properly. They don't complete a course of medication sometimes; they just stop taking it when the symptoms go away, so a week later they're back in the hospital. Or they double the dose in order to get better twice as fast. That sort of thing. And that's with a system of regulation through prescriptions.

M: So the point of regulation is to protect them against making serious errors in the use of drugs?

C: Yes, to protect them.

M: But doesn't that violate your principle that people have autonomy over their bodies? Shouldn't you let them take whatever they please if you are really a believer in that principle?

C: Well, I do believe in that principle. But I guess it isn't the only principle I believe in. Sometimes there is a question of protecting people's interests, their health, even their lives. Like treating an unconscious patient who comes into emergency. You can't bother about consent or autonomy there. That doesn't mean you don't believe in autonomy as a principle. But in that situation it just can't come into account.

M: Yes, I see. So the principle that you seem to be using is that sometimes a person's autonomy can be restricted or overridden, when there is some important good to be gained that way. Like saving an unconscious patient, or protecting someone from misusing drugs, or deceiving Mr. Angstimmer in the ICU.

C: Yes.

M: Is it a question of beneficence, of doing some good?

C: Yes.

M: Then why isn't your position on abortion vulnerable on the same grounds? That is, why can't the right to make decisions about one's body be overridden here on the ground that some good will result for the child?

C: That just isn't the same. In the other cases—the unconscious patient or the patient who wants to take a lot of powerful drugs—we're just helping that person. We're restricting him, or doing something to him, that he would *want* us to do if he were conscious or if he were reasonable. But if you prohibit abortion, then you are preventing a woman from doing what she wants to do. You're not doing her any good at all.

M: I understand, yes. Perhaps there is a clear position here. Do I have it right? You respect people's autonomy over their own bodies except when you have to limit it for their own good?

C: Right.

M: And that's why we can restrict drugs—that protects people from their own errors. But we can't prohibit abortion because that limitation does not protect people from their own errors.

C: Yes.

M: And I suppose that is why we don't want to let people sell their bodily organs. When the rich man who needs a kidney transplant is willing to pay a large sum of money, and the poor man would be willing to sell a kidney, we step in and say, "That is no good, that we won't allow." And you would agree?

C: Yes, I would. That protects the poor man against damaging himself because of the financial problems. We have to have a voluntary system for organs.

M: Now what about the flasher—the guy who exposes himself outside the window of the women's dormitory or on a busy shopping street?

C: What about him? I'm not following your reasoning here.

M: We restrict him; we try to prevent that behavior. Shouldn't we?

C: Of course we should.

M: But isn't he just doing what he wants to do with his body? Or the guy who takes off all his clothes on a hot day so he can sunbathe in a public park?

C: That's a different matter. These people are socially deviant; the behavior is just not accepted in society. They're probably in need of treatment.

M: But are they always? Suppose the nude sunbather just believes that society is too rigid and repressive about nudity. And he likes the sun. So it is a form of social protest. He takes off his clothes as a way of saying that we should accept the human body without shame or embarrassment, that we should change our values. Do we prevent him? It isn't obvious that he is in need of treatment.

C: Yes, we prevent him because that sort of behavior is so upsetting to others. Maybe he is even right in principle. But until that attitude is accepted, then his behavior is disruptive and upsetting to other people. And some would say damaging, psychologically damaging, to children, who are not prepared to handle it.

M: So we seem to have a second reason for limiting a person's autonomy over his body. We can limit it when that person's behavior is damaging to someone else.

C: Sometimes we have to. To protect others.

M: And if public nudity could be shown to be really very damaging, that would make the case even stronger against it?

C: It would have to.

M: What if—this takes some stretch of the imagination—what if some people would actually drop dead at the sight of public nudity? A small percentage of the population with a particular genetic disease. Show them genitalia in public, and they fall over dead just like that. Then what would you say about public nudity?

C: That would make it more serious, not just a nuisance.

M: So we would have to limit the nudist's freedom to do with his body as he pleases because otherwise, there would be serious damage to others, including loss of life?

C: Yes.

M: Then you seem to have come around to Dr. Healer's position. To protect the right to life of other people, we sometimes have to limit what someone can do with his or her own body. Isn't the prohibition of abortion a clear case of that?

H: I knew philosophy would be on my side. There's no way out of that reasoning.

C: I don't know. I don't know what to say, but I'm not comfortable about it. It just doesn't seem right to me.

M: Well, why don't you think about it for a while? Because I want to take a closer look at Dr. Healer's argument. I'm not so ready as he is to judge which side philosophy is on.

H: But didn't you just show that I was right?

M: No, all I showed was that there are problems with Dr. Care's argument. Now let's have a look at yours. Do you think every woman is obligated to have children?

H: No, of course not. Most women want children. But I don't say they have to have them or want them. Why?

M: I'm recalling your remark that you cannot will that your mother should have had an abortion. Can you will that your mother should have chosen not to have children at all, not to have become pregnant in the first place?

H: I don't see how I can. That would come to the same thing: no me.

M: I agree. But you do think your mother had a right to decide for herself whether or not she wanted to have children?

H: Yes, of course. It is just good for me that she decided to.

M: Then I think that's the end of your argument. You can't will that your mother should have had an abortion. Neither can you will that she should have decided not to have children. But she had a right to decide not to have children. So why didn't she have a right, also, to decide to have an abortion?

H: I see, I see. It isn't just a question of what I can will. Okay. But they're still not the same. Deciding not to have a child doesn't violate anybody's right to life. There isn't anybody whose right is violated. But if a woman is pregnant, then an abortion violates that specific baby's right to life. So I can deny that my mother had a right to an abortion, just as I deny that any mother has a right to an abortion.

M: All right. We've filtered out the part about what you can will. So let's have a closer look at the question of the right to life. I notice that the language you use is interesting. You said in your original argument that *others* have the same right to life that you claim for yourself and that you deny that *mothers* have a right to an abortion. And just now you spoke of a *baby's* right to life. Doesn't that seem a bit tendentious?

H: What do you mean?

M: I mean this. If a pregnant woman is considering an abortion, especially in a very early stage of pregnancy, she may think it makes a great deal of difference whether the life in question is that of another person or not. Compare these two sentences: First, "*A* mother has no right to terminate the life of her baby; that violates another's right to life." And second, "*A* woman has no right to terminate the life of her fetus; that violates a fetus's right to life." The first sentence is justified only if a fetus is another person with a right to life. The second sentence puts the issue in a more neutral way. I'm just suggesting that your use of terms like *mother*, *other*, and *baby* is a way of prejudging some of the basic questions.

H: Yes, I see that. But I don't see that it matters much. Because the second sentence is enough. I'll stand on that way of putting it.

M: But that may not be so easy. You see, we all agree that others have a right to life. And we all understand that if a woman is a mother, there must be a child whose mother she is. So if we accept the language of the first sentence, we have already accepted a lot of important substance. But the second sentence is not persuasive. Why does a woman have no right to terminate the life of her fetus?

H: Because it violates the fetus's right to life.

M: Why do you think a fetus has a right to life?

H: Because everyone has. You just said that yourself, and you said we all agree to it.

M: No, you're not listening carefully enough. What I said we all agree to is that others—meaning other persons—have a right to life. Now you are claiming that fetuses have a right to life because everyone—that is, every person—has such a right. But that only follows on the assumption that fetuses are persons.

H: Yes, I see the logic. But it is no problem for my argument. Of course, I consider the fetus to be a person. That's the whole point.

M: Suppose I don't agree that the fetus is a person? You won't convince me simply by asserting that it is.

H: No. But if you agree that children are persons, then you have a problem. You have to explain how you decide when to count that developing entity— whatever you want to call it—as a person. And the best answer is the time of conception. That's the only sensible answer.

C: That isn't so clear. There's a policy decision about what to count as a person, and no argument that just rests on the assertion that there is a person right from the start can succeed. So I'm right after all; a woman has a right to an abortion because that doesn't violate anybody else's rights. There isn't anybody else in the story yet.

H: Even at eight months? Or nine? That's absurd.

C: I didn't say that. But at least at the beginning.

M: Now hold on. Let's not jump to conclusions. Maybe this is a good time to review what has happened so far. We haven't shown anybody to be right yet. All we've done is look at each of the two arguments and discover that neither one is really adequate, neither one is convincing. But neither of you is shown to be right just because the other one's argument has flaws.

C: But where do we go from here?

H: And how do we deal with the disagreement that remains?

M: That won't be easy. It may not even be possible. But we can see what the possibilities are. It will depend, among other things, on how wedded you are to the positions you started with. If you, Dr. Care, are unwilling to abandon your support for abortion on demand, no matter what the arguments, then your position is more like a creed than a conclusion, and it won't matter where the reasoning leads. And if you, Dr. Healer, are determined to remain totally opposed to abortion no matter what, then you, too, will be simply standing firm on a dogmatic position, and reasons won't have any bearing.

H: No, it isn't like that. I want to do what is right, to support the view that is right. It isn't just that I'm comfortable in terms of my background with an antiabortion view or that I believe it blindly. I've held that view because I am convinced that it is right. I think I could change my position if the arguments against it were stronger than those for it. But nobody has convinced me of that. I do admit to being upset by the flaws in my argument. I guess I just never thought about it carefully enough.

C: I agree with that. I mean, I never meant to give the impression that I thought abortion was a trivial or frivolous matter. I want to stand on the right position, too. And that leads me to defend freedom of choice. But I think I could modify my position if I saw really good evidence that a different position was better.

M: Then we've done what we can for now. We haven't resolved any of these three disputes, of course. And it may be that in the end your differences will be irreconcilable. But nothing I've heard so far convinces me that they must be. I'm sure you both realize that I do not speak for all of philosophy. And I've tried to refrain from offering substantive views of my own. Instead, I've tried to help you become clearer about your own positions and the reasons you can give to defend them and to help you have a somewhat more sympathetic understanding of each other's views. Our discussion has had to be fairly superficial in such a short time. Still, you've both shown that in addition to some very obvious disagreements, you do share a substantial basis for further discussions and possibly for some resolution.

The point of this dialogue is to illustrate that philosophical inquiry into the reasons behind conflicting moral judgments can facilitate resolution of the conflict by placing those reasons in the broader context of shared values. I do not claim it can always be done, but I dispute MacIntyre's claim that it can never be done—that we are literally resourceless. One reason why it might be impossible in a given case is that a common moral ground may indeed be absent and unachievable. Still, if philosophy can help find the common ground where it does or can exist—as is surely true in many difficult cases—then there is much that physicians, patients, and citizens can reasonably expect from moral philosophy. Of course, on my account there will be unresolved conflict and enduring moral uncertainty. I simply do not ask that moral philosophy eliminate moral dilemma before I will acknowledge it as useful and important. I am willing to respect it for what it can do instead of lamenting what it cannot.

Virtues can indeed become vices; the prolongation of life is a case in point. That traditional medical value has become more problematic both because of our increased ability to prolong life in the face of an unhappy prognosis and because of our increased understanding of why it is that life is valuable. The physician does face tragic dilemmas, for example, in dealing with the tenuous lives of certain patients with grave congenital defects. What makes the physician's dilemma tragic is the profound seriousness of making a mistake. Yet the sense of tragedy can be over-done. Virtue does not lie in saintliness any more than knowledge lies in certainty. Physicians can act with moral integrity even in the face of moral uncertainty, although doing so adds new demands to those of medical competence.

Philosophy can help articulate those new demands and help point the way toward meeting them. It can help us understand the relations between our actions and our aspirations and can teach us to accept as necessary the moral conflict that inevitably arises from the clash between what we want and what the world will yield to us. It can help us identify and understand what we really do value. Moreover, philosophy to some extent can provide a positive moral theory based on the moral content of our pluralistic culture. In sum, it can tell us not, as MacIntyre claims, why we cannot hope for solutions "in a culture which precisely lacks the means to solve moral problems," but rather what sorts of solutions we can reasonably hope for. And it can help guide us toward them. Of course, moral philosophy alone cannot provide solutions to moral problems any more than law alone can eliminate legal problems or economics alone can eliminate economic problems. We must always reach beyond philosophy in addressing problems in the world. But we should be wary of reaching without it.

MacIntyre writes that "what matters most in a period in which human life is tragic is to have the strength to resist false solutions." No period of human history has been devoid of tragedy; none, I'm sure, ever will be. Human life is always partly tragic, and false solutions should always be resisted. So, too, should false despair. This more optimistic view is shared by Nagel, who acknowledges the inevitability of conflict between moral perspectives, but who then goes on to write:

Does this mean, then, that basic practical conflicts have no solution? The unavailability of a single, reductive method or a clear set of priorities for settling them does not remove the necessity for making decisions in such cases. When faced with conflicting and incommensurable claims we still have to do something—even if it is only to do nothing. And the fact that action must be unitary seems to imply that unless justification is also unitary, nothing can be either right or wrong and all decisions under conflict are arbitrary.

I believe this is wrong, but the alternative is hard to explain. Briefly, I contend that there can be good judgment without total justification, either explicit or implicit. The fact that one cannot say why a certain decision is the correct one, given a particular balance of conflicting reasons, does not mean that the claim to correctness is meaningless. Provided one has taken the process of practical justification as far as it will go in the course of arriving at the conflict, one may be able to proceed without further justification, but without irrationality, either. What makes this possible is *judgment*—essentially the faculty Aristotle described as practical wisdom, which reveals itself over time in individual decisions rather than in the enunciation of general principles. It will not always yield a solution: there are true practical dilemmas that have no solution, and there are also conflicts so complex that judgment cannot operate confidently. But in many cases it can be relied on to take up the slack that remains beyond the limits of explicit rational argument.[1]

Moreover, our pluralistic culture is not as fragmentary as it can appear, and moral guidance can be found to some extent in its hidden coherence. For despite the apparently stark incompatibility among the various moral theories we have glimpsed, they share certain common characteristics that constitute a core of agreement about moral judgment—a common denominator that lies at the heart of our moral outlook despite its diversity. Each theory satisfies the condition that as moral agents all persons are equal and subject to the same fundamental constraints and entitlements that limit moral action for anyone else. This principle of universalizability sets our moral outlook apart from those that endorse hierarchical or caste systems of moral standing. And each of these moral theories is based on a respect for persons—for their rights, interests, and aspirations in different degrees, to be sure—but a respect all the same, that sets our moral outlook apart from those that place the individual in a position of servitude to the interests of a source of value—be it political, theological, or otherwise—that supersedes individual persons in moral importance.

These are independent points about this collection of moral perspectives; a moral theory could satisfy either one alone. That is, a theory could treat all persons alike, but not in a manner that is based on respect for persons. This would be true of a theory for which equality was a basic value, although service to the state was the overriding good to which the rights and interests of individuals, all of them equally, could be sacrificed. Another theory could hold that the source of all value lies in the interests of individual people, although the interests of some people—the more noble and worthy among humankind—are endowed with greater moral importance. Neither of these theories would stand up well under sustained scrutiny. On the contrary, that they each lack one of the two characteristics we are considering would justify their rejection. They serve here only to demonstrate that these two characteristics are genuinely independent and that they are each substantively significant.

These characteristics limit moral choice in the face of conflict. They provide a backdrop that gives our moral outlook a distinguishable stamp. That outlook is not fragmentary in a random way but has a logic that emerges from amidst the pluralism. People are complex, value many things, and do so in ways that distinguish one person from another. Because our deepest commitments are to equality and to respect for persons as moral agents and as the possessors of interests, feelings, and aspirations, we respect a diversity of approaches to closing the gap between what the contending moral theories collectively allow and what in the end one chooses to do. Choice is not entirely unconstrained, for we condemn actions that violate our commitment to equality (such as denying voting rights to the poor) or to respect for persons (such as punishing an innocent man when it would be socially useful, claiming his interests do not count). But the moral common denominators that we can identify still leave unresolved questions about the adjudication of moral conflict.

Faced with such a conflict, an individual must make a choice, and that choice will constitute an exercise of moral judgment. How one responds to such situations is an important ingredient in one's character and personality—a source of diversity in action that we are bound to respect by virtue of our commitment to respect for persons as moral agents. Thus, insofar as respect for persons is a justifiable value, a certain amount of pluralism in ethical perspective is a sign not of moral decay, but of moral progress, of our transcending the strictures of moral hegemony to achieve a respect for persons that allows them the freedom to exercise moral judgment—sometimes well and sometimes perhaps less well—as they pursue their individual objectives and interests. Only when their choices violate the basic commitments to universalizability or to respect for persons can we condemn their actions as definitively and demonstrably wrong. But as their actions unfold over time, some will emerge as having exercised a quality of moral judgment that merits admiration, and others will emerge as self-serving, deceptive, or unfair and will be judged accordingly.

Respect for persons and for equality can take many forms, and bitter conflict as well as searing uncertainty will never be dispelled, especially from an undertaking, like clinical medicine, that is permeated with the need to make decisions that affect human interests so deeply. The more one understands the factors that are relevant to moral choice, the greater the likelihood that one's judgment will bear the test of scrutiny over time. Such understanding is not easily acquired, however, in part because it is so difficult to characterize, but for other reasons also. In a later chapter I will offer some conjectures on how such understanding can be made more likely; I will do so in the context of discussing what is involved in being a good doctor.

At the level of social policy, closure is no easier to attain than at the level of individual decision. It is sometimes achievable, as when there is widespread public agreement about a question that began as controversial. This is close to the case now with respect to fluoridation of the water supply, a practice which is generally accepted but was at one time bitterly opposed by a significant constituency. But at other times closure on the substantive issue in dispute is out of reach. That surely is, and will remain, the case in regard to abortion policy; it is the case, but one day may cease to be so, in the debate about nuclear power. When a moral conflict emerges at the level of public policy, and when closure on the substance of the issue seems impossible, a different sort of closure can be sought, however. Where we all cannot be satisfied with a decision that is made, we can at least try to fashion a process for making it that brings the dispute to rest fairly, having incorporated respectful consideration of the views of all interested parties. Whatever decision results will displease some, but that cannot be avoided when opinion is sharply divided about what the outcome should be. The process can nonetheless gain the respect of the public by ensuring that the judgment in the end is based on a conscientious assessment of the full range of relevant factors.

At the level of individual decisions, however, we search in vain for a procedural analogue. Precisely the difference between a decision faced by an individual and a matter of public or social choice is that there is no collective responsibility or involvement in the individual choice. The physician in the fertility clinic could consult with his colleagues about what to do, and he could call for the formal adoption of a clinic policy toward cases of the sort that he faced, but even prior to that he has to confront, alone, the need to provide an initial response to the woman's request. And in the subsequent deliberations with colleagues, he would still face, alone, the need to determine what his position would be in the ensuing debate about a collective viewpoint. Individual choice thus requires the exercise of moral judgment in a more fundamental way than collective choice. And the only way to ensure that it is based on a full consideration of the morally relevant factors is for the individual who faces the decision to be aware of those factors and disposed to take them respectfully into account.

In the next section we will consider a few specific issues in medicine and health policy. In each case we will explore the way conceptual clarity can lead toward a deeper understanding of the decisions that have to be made, whether it be the physician, the patient, the policymaker, or the citizen who faces the choice. In the penultimate chapter, we will return to our starting point—the behavior of the physician—in order to examine what constitutes being a good doctor and how it can be made more likely that doctors will satisfy the standard I will propose. Although that standard is stated in the context of characterizing the good doctor, its ingredients exemplify moral conscientiousness more generally. That chapter may thus be viewed as a discussion of learning to make morally sound choices, whatever the role we fill.

PART THREE

Selected Topics

9
Dealing with Dying

I WANT NOW to consider in more detail some of the moral issues related to medical treatment of the dying. In particular, I will seek some clarity about what dying is, who counts as doing it, and whether it makes sense to fear death, to seek to avoid it, and to lament it when it comes to others. My concern is with those who are dying and with some of the circumstances surrounding them. Such persons, of course, are very much alive. Still, I do need to focus some attention on the subject of death since it is death that gives dying its special poignancy.

A death can occur too soon or too late. Further, there is the question of how it will come about. There are dyings that are slow and agonizing and dyings that are gentle and graceful. It's the latter sort to which one aspires, but there is a substantial risk of being overtaken by froward circumstances. It seems reasonable that if death is impending, one should want to exert some influence on the mode of one's dying. Just as one wants to be able to influence the major events that shape and constitute a life at earlier stages, one may want to avoid the indignity of having to witness and endure a final stage not as an effective agent, but merely a deteriorating object.

A death will come too soon if one has, as it approaches, aspirations and projects which engage one's interest and endow one's ongoing life with purpose. As the distinguished British philosopher Bernard Williams has noted, "To want something . . . is to that extent to have a reason for resisting what excludes having that thing; and death certainly does that, for a very large range of things that one wants."[1] It is reasonable to view one's own death as an evil so long as one is up to something

[153]

one cares about with which it will interfere. Death may be no evil to the dead, but it can still be an evil to the living.

On the other hand, one's death comes too late if lacking aspirations and projects that carry one forward, life drags on devoid of the point that only one's purposes could give it. So there are two distinct respects in which one's dying can go awry. One may do it in a bad way, and one may do it at a bad time.

This sense of a well-timed death arises in part from a biographical sense of life—that is, of the life that each person leads. It is not grandiose for people to consider their lives as biographies in the making. Every life *is* a biography in the making, even though most are of limited public interest and, at the hands of most biographers, not worth writing. This sense of one's life can be overdone, as when one begins to act for the sake of the story, choosing what to do primarily on the basis of what would make the best literary material. Still, our aesthetic sense has a place here. In assessing a life about which we are reading, we may judge that the life, overall, was less happy or noble or valuable than it might otherwise have been because it ended badly. And our sense of a bad ending is not merely based on simplistic considerations of whether there was pain in the dying or whether aspirations were left unfulfilled. Our sense of a bad ending involves our sense of the story as a whole. For Hemingway to die by his own hand in the face of physical deterioration seems fitting in a way in which other suicides may not be. One may quite reasonably desire that the story of one's life not be a tragic tale and that it be a tale rich with character development, coherence of plot, and other literary virtues—including an ending that makes sense, in both mode and moment, in the context of what has gone before.

This way of contemplating a life has an advantage: It helps us achieve a valuable detachment from our usual absorption in living. Such detachment is essential for our being able to take stock of our lives in order to exercise judgment about and reasoned influence on the shapes our lives take.

Ortega y Gasset claimed: "Life is of no consequence if a formidable eagerness to widen its frontiers does not stamp within its confines."[2] For some of us, his observation strikes a responsive chord. Yet even if we accept such a criterion of having consequences as being applicable to our own lives, we must be wary of imposing it on others. What will make another person's life have consequence for him will depend on the sorts of projects and aspirations that he has. The more they differ from our own, the harder it is to identify with that person, but the difficulty should not incline us to impose more familiar and comfortable criteria of meaningfulness on other people's lives. It follows that our judgment about the ending of another person's life cannot be well made without some knowledge of the story of that life.

If we know enough about that story, we may see the final stage—the dying—as nothing to combat before the fact or lament after the fact, nor its mode appropriate to alter. The dying may be proceeding just as its subject would have it, given the constraints imposed by the physical and social worlds. It is possible for me to see the death and the dying of another as no evils for that person and to refuse to lament them on that other's account—not from any insouciance, but because there is nothing to lament. At the same time I may sorely grieve my own loss in the other's death—for my interest in another's life may be substantially different from his. For example, I may have a deep emotional dependence on a woman whose life, my dependence on it notwithstanding, holds no point or prospects for her. Or I may be the agent of a writer whose death is a good one in the context of her total life story, but which at the same time deals me a severe economic blow. Or—more to the point—I may be a physician attending a patient whose death, welcome and benign from the patient's point of view, aggravates my anxiety, erodes my ego, and sullies my statistics. But if I have no vested interest in the other's life, no reason for valuing its continuation, and if its continuation has no value for that other, then it is hard to see why its continuation should be thought to have any value at all. If we simply *assume* that it must have value, it may be of use to become clear about whose purposes and needs give rise to that assumption.

I am not suggesting that anyone's dying should be taken lightly. On the contrary, I am saying that if we take a person's dying seriously, as we would a person's education, marriage, or career, then we must consider it that person's own, unique dying, the final stage of a particular life. To consider it thus is to require of ourselves that we see it in the context of the story of that life, not merely as one more instance of a general evil. It is far easier, of course, simply to dig in on the side of life and repel the repugnant reaper however we can.

But do we clearly understand just what the reaper represents? What constitutes death is not a fact to discover, but a decision to make. We easily identify clear cases of life—such as a person actively engaged in some familiar enterprise—and of death—such as the decaying remains of a former person. In between we can find hard cases. It was once thought that if anything was hard about cases at the border it was to discover whether, as a matter of empirical fact, the vital forces or substance had departed quite yet, or merely seemed to have. Now we can know what is physiologically true of a patient without knowing whether or not to call that patient dead. When we seek a definition of death to help resolve the status of a patient, we find that we must test each possible definition against an independent judgment about whether we wish to classify people in such circumstances as dead or alive. So we cannot look to definitions to decide the hard cases; we must decide the case as part of the process of fashioning and testing the definition. The kind of case often cited to illustrate the point is that of the patient with severe, irreversible damage to the neocortex, who sustains enough brain-stem function to maintain spontaneous circulatory and respiratory activity indefinitely in total absence of consciousness or any prospect of consciousness. What shall we decide of such a case?

A substantial literature surrounds the issue. I will emphasize just one aspect of the debate that is apposite. The definition of death that we endorse reflects our reasons for valuing life. If we hold that it is only experiences that have intrinsic value, then it is plain why life is precious. Life is the precondition of experience and hence is necessary for all else that has value. But this view, while accounting for the preciousness of life, bases that preciousness on the connection between life, which has instrumental value, and the experience it makes possible, which alone can have intrinsic value. Where there is no experience or prospect of experience, life loses its luster. In the case at issue we may say that the biologically viable organism, devoid irreversibly of sentience, has life that is no longer of value and that we may thus abandon with impunity. And the device by which we abandon life that has no value may be to declare death. Thus, a criterion of death based on neocortical function reflects our prior judgment that life without it, and hence without experience, is devoid of value and so a sort of death.

But if we hold that life itself has intrinsic value, entirely apart from experience, then the question of sentience does not arise. The irrevocably comatose are nonetheless alive, despite their lack of sentience, and their lives, having the value that inheres in all human life, must be sustained. No definition or criterion of death in terms of neocortical activity will do. Our patient is alive after all and thus qualifies for care.

Our conceptions of value are thus intertwined with our criteria for classifying cases. As medical intervention more subtly, sensitively, and selectively separates the complex farrago of functions that constitute a fully living person, we see emerging a continuum of states that ranges from the clearly living to the clearly dead through those who are alive in some ways and dead in others. How we want to relate to the mixed and marginal cases determines what we take death to be, and the moral and conceptual issues are not separable.

The search for an operational definition of death is motivated largely by the desire to fashion guidelines for the resolution of clinical quandaries. Which definition of death is adopted can have immediate consequences, sometimes of a dramatic sort. Either the kidney is made available in time for the lifesaving transplant, or it is not. Either the intravenous feeding continues and the patient is kept in a bed, or it stops and the corpse is put in a coffin. Either the family lingers on in an indeterminate agony of resignation beyond hope or hope beyond reason, or the family shifts to the patterns of behavior appropriate to mourning its loss. It is no wonder a palatable definition of death is earnestly sought.

Lost in that search is the fact that we also classify people at various times as dying. Little attention has been paid to what it means to speak of someone as dying, yet this too has behavioral consequences. They are not the decisive and dramatic consequences associated with disputes over definitions of death. Yet, in subtler ways, how we think of what dying is affects how we treat and relate to people. Let us shift the focus to dying.

Life in full flower is an ongoing actualization of possibilities. Even Oblomov, to whom action was anathema, was carried forward from one moment to the next by deliberations about the possibilities before him, and the constant reaffirmation of his indecisiveness became a mode of acting that gave his life its special stamp. Dying closes off possibilities. Human relationships consist in a shared actualizing of possibilities available for choice. Dying thus transforms relationships, replacing the sense of future that nourishes them with a sense of ending that tends to impoverish them. So it matters whether or not one is classified as dying.

Stalin is reputed to have replied to inquiry about a rumored fatal illness, "Of course I am dying. I have been since the day I was born." We all are dying in this sense, synonymous with *mortal*, that makes no distinctions among us. But we must seek an account of *dying* that captures the sense of that term which is associated with *impending* death as opposed to *eventual* death. Again, we can readily identify clear cases. Ivan Ilyich, in Tolstoy's "The Death of Ivan Ilyich,"[3] on his penultimate day is dying; Hans Castorp, as his journey to the mountains begins, in Thomas Mann's *The Magic Mountain*,[4] is not. In between, it is a matter of some dispute.

What are the conditions under which it is correct to say that someone is dying? We can approach the question by reminding ourselves of what sorts of circumstances lead us to think of someone as dying. The paradigmatic cases in fashionable forums on fatality seem to be the terminally ill adult, diagnosed as having a short but indeterminate life expectancy, whose physician isn't sure about what to tell him, and a pain-racked or insensate patient at the brink of death, whose physician is unsure about whether or how long to try to sustain life. But the dying are not necessarily aged or diseased; they include the injured, the young, and perhaps those whose plight is more a function of circumstances than of health, such as trapped miners or divers. Is there anything they all have in common?

As a first approximation to an answer, I suggest that a person who has a generally irreversible illness or pattern of deterioration or is inextricably in circumstances known to lead to and cause death soon is dying. This analysis, of course, stands in need of further explication and refinement. But it does not matter at all whether this account is correct in detail; what is important is only that the correct account will be like this one in certain respects. Any refinement of the above account would have to clarify such notions as those of dying *soon* or of what is *irreversible* or *inextricable*. The account depends essentially on these elusive notions, and if I am right, any correct account of what dying is must share that dependency.

What these notions have in common is their judgmental quality. What counts as dying soon can never be measured by an EEG; we decide what counts as imminent in part on the basis of how we want to treat and relate to people in various circumstances. We decide what are inextricable circumstances in part on the basis of what our priorities are for allocating resources. And so on. Thus, we decide who the dying are not merely on the basis of discoverable medical fact but also on the basis of value-laden judgments that are presupposed by our conceptions of what it is to be dying.

It is commonly assumed that since dying is simply approaching death, what counts as dying will be determined once it is resolved what is to count as death. I have argued that this is simply not so—that even given agreement about what constitutes death, the way we classify people as dying is value-laden.

Those who are judged to be dying are often in, or about to be in, the hands of providers of medical treatment. Note the variety of ways in which physicians and their associates can relate to dying persons.

The first relationship is diagnostic, primarily the physician is the one who typically classifies a patient as dying. If the patient's condition is bad enough, the physician may classify him, instead, as already having died, in which case the function is one of pronouncement and certification, rather than of diagnosis or treatment. If the patient is diagnosed as dying, the most common relationship between the physician and the patient is that of immediate medical intervention aimed at forestalling death—at holding it at bay for as long as possible. Sometimes, however, the physician relinquishes resistance and acquiesces in the arrival of death, shifting the focus from the patient's survival to the patient's physical comfort. The physician may even facilitate the ending by withdrawing certain treatments or by making the means of suicide available. In extreme cases the physician may go beyond facilitating death, actively intervening to terminate the life in his care.

These functions—judging, forestalling, facilitating, and terminating—are the most obvious medical functions in relation to dying. But the responsibilities of medicine include other functions. The increased ability of medical intervention to forestall death seems to have overshadowed the function of dealing supportively with the living problems of the dying patient. It is one benefit of the recent popularity of death as a topic that some redress of this imbalance is well under way.[5] Work of the kind exemplified by the early efforts of Dr. Kübler-Ross and in the hospice movement demonstrates the value of striving to serve the needs of dying patients.[6] Finally, the physician bears a responsibility for dealing with those problems of survivors that relate to the dying and death of others—of attending to the aftermath of death. Let us consider each of the six functions in turn.

I have argued that the judgmental function is not simply a matter of application of scientific or medical expertise but depends on evaluative assumptions that different persons might not share. A patient, assuming he knows the medical facts that are true of him, might consider himself to be dying, as judged from the perspective of his life story and the values that infuse it; his physician, perhaps unaware of the patient's aspirations and priorities for resource allocation, may not perceive the patient as dying. Insofar as the "dying" label changes one's sense of the possibilities or influences the way others perceive and relate to one, the difference in judgment between the physician and the patient can underlie a difference about how the patient should be treated. Of course, insofar as the patient is unable to make an informed judgment on the issue, because of ignorance of the medical facts or for other reasons, his ability to participate autonomously in decisions about his treatment is curtailed.

The moral problems associated with forestalling death are more obvious. The usual list includes: the question of the justifiability of using extended exotic therapies to forestall the death of a patient whose prospects for life are tenebrous at best; the question of the relevance of economic considerations to decisions about whether, how, and for how long to attempt to forestall death; and the question of the extent to which others than the dying have obligations to participate in the effort to forestall death, e.g., by donating blood or a kidney. There are other questions as well. Pervading them all is the more fundamental question of whether death is always an evil to be combated or whether under some conditions a more accepting posture is appropriate. The debates about suicide, euthanasia, and death with dignity begin at this point.

Facilitating death seems at first to be an intermediate relationship somewhere between accepting death and causing it. Applying the concept, however, is not always easy. In a famous case at Johns Hopkins Hospital, a Down's Syndrome baby with duodenal atresia, whose life could have been saved by surgery had the parents allowed it, died instead after many days in the hospital without food or medical treatment.[7] In the debate that followed public disclosure of that case, some argued that the hospital personnel simply let the baby die. Others held that the baby was killed, no less than had it been injected with potassium chloride—though perhaps less mercifully. If facilitating death lies between letting it happen and causing it, it is hard to make much sense of the notion in cases like this.

If a normal child with a curable infection dies because the antibiotic was withheld either inadvertently or deliberately, we view that withholding as having culpably caused the death. If the child is instead an extremely damaged newborn with no significant prospects for survival, we are more inclined to see a similar withholding as simple noninterference with benign natural processes. If the patient is in the late stages of an excruciating terminal illness, the decision not to treat may be viewed as facilitating imminent death, as might the intended administration of a high enough dosage of analgesic to suppress respiration.

Philosophers sometimes question the reality of what others take for granted. Sometimes such arguments strike the plain man as fantasy. But the philosopher's skepticism cannot always be easily dismissed. Physicians and others often do accept as legitimate, clear, and important the ostensible distinctions among killing, facilitating death, and letting die. Thus, the organization Concern for Dying argues for passive euthanasia—an intended allowing to die under certain circumstances—while explicitly not advocating active euthanasia—the intentional intervention to terminate life.[8] And troubled physicians sometimes find solace in the thought that whereas they could never be a party to deliberate termination of life, a humane acceptance of the approach of death requires that they let some patients die by refraining from providing treatment. But other physicians are less comfortable with these distinctions.

Here the philosopher's skepticism may find its mark. The arguments are strong that acts of omission are as significant causally and morally as their more visible counterparts, the acts of commission.[9] If I can prevent your death by giving you the antidote to a poison you have inadvertently taken, it is hard to see how my deliberate refraining from doing so can be distinguished morally from my giving you poison in the first place. But unless some such distinction can be made out, the physician who allows a patient to die, in peace and dignity or in any other way, when the means of forestalling death were available, may be indulging himself in a deception—comforting, perhaps, but a deception still—when he believes his behavior is morally different from active euthanasia. (I do not deny that the consequences of a social policy that encourages active euthanasia might be very different from those of one that discourages it.)

Some people take the difficulty of distinguishing among allowing, facilitating, and causing death to constitute a part of the argument in favor of making every effort to forestall death. Others use the same point in support of active euthanasia. Thus, the issues surrounding the termination of life are inseparable from those surrounding allowing or facilitating death.

The function of caring supportively for the dying patient raises different kinds of concerns. Nobody likes to invest in a losing proposition, and dying persons are losing propositions from many points of view. Emotional capital is limited, for health care providers as well as for everyone else. There seems to be no long-term payoff from investing it in dying strangers. It is thus no surprise that once a person is viewed as dying, the inclination to care for that person declines markedly. The induration faced by dying persons in hospitals is particularly well reported of late; it is in hospitals, most of all, that dying is an affront to one's hosts and hence is socially unacceptable behavior.

This familiar pattern of withdrawal from the dying is primarily self-protective. Dying persons are nonetheless persons for their dying, and their need to sustain satisfying relationships is nonetheless intense for their circumstances being discomforting. For most of us, the usual patterns of relating to others are primarily predicated on the existence of future-oriented, ongoing possibilities. To the extent that the dying person faces a truncated future, those patterns of relating to people seem awkward, disingenuous, or even impossible. Yet respect for the present needs of dying persons demands the fashioning of patterns of relating to them on terms that make sense for them. That requires going beyond the treatment of their pain and of their bodies. It requires at times the courage to join with them in an acknowledgment of their plight, legitimizing and participating in their efforts to come to terms with that plight.

Once a patient has died, attending to the aftermath frequently involves a physician, almost as an automatic consequence of his role as the one who certifies death and reports it to survivors. Once the death certificate is signed, the sedatives commonly follow close behind. Immediate reactions of shock, grief, relief, guilt, and all the rest that are bound up with confronting the death of someone close are obvious and become the focus of medical care. Yet here we see an ironic reversal. The focus of attention on the dying person tends to be on the body—the physical organism, with respect to which the physician has a repertoire of techniques of intervention. The emotional needs of the dying person are slighted, and thus, we note the present campaign to reestablish an awareness of the living humanity of persons approaching death. Yet as soon as one turns from the dying patient to the survivors, psychological sensitivity reasserts itself, almost as if, no longer repressed by the minatory prospect of dealing with death, it is relieved at the chance to face less intimidating problems like grief or shock. Yet just as dying persons have minds as well as bodies, survivors have bodies as well as minds, and their bodies are placed in greater jeopardy by the stress of their loss.

The mortality rate for survivors of a death is markedly greater than for populations otherwise similar.[10] This effect can be seen both in humans and in other species. Creatures do die of grief and other stressful emotions that often accompany bereavement. Thus, it is statistically true that the physical well-being of the survivors of a death is eroded by that death. In a given case, of course, this effect may be wholly lacking; the merry widow's dalliance may begin to the strains of the dirge. The extent to which a given survivor's health is undermined by the death will depend in part on the role the deceased had played in the survivor's life. Knowing something of the story of that life thus may be an essential part of being able to attend responsibly to the aftermath of the death. In the days of the family physician, such familiarity with the special circumstances of survivors was expected. Now the deceased's oncologist, for example, may play a minor role in meeting the survivor's needs, and the survivor's own medical care may be in the hands of disparate specialists or an impersonal clinic or, in the absence of symptoms at the time of the death, in no hands at all. Thus, certain aspects of attending to the aftermath of a death may get scant consideration, in part in consequence of the structure of modern health care delivery.

The irreversibility of death gives those situations that involve it a reverberating gravity. Thus, in dealing with dying, one faces strict standards if moral integrity is to be maintained. Conscientiousness in such situations involves acknowledging that the approaching death can be judged only in the context of the story of the life that it will end, and that context involves the patient's beliefs and attitudes as much as his physiological characteristics. The conscientious physician will have the courage to face his own feelings about death, the honesty to distinguish between his own interest in the patient's life and the patient's interest in that life, and the concern to invest the requisite time and effort to understand enough of the story of that life to participate in decisions in an informed way.[11] Even then the physician dealing with a dying patient cannot be certain of acting fully in accord with the values that will bear scrutiny on reflection; more likely there will be regret from time to time. Accepting one's own moral missteps, however—acknowledging and learning from them with neither arrogance nor defeatism—is also an aspect of moral integrity.

The physician, then, even without standards of morality that can conclusively resolve all the dilemmas that arise, can still adopt as a morally compelling objective the goal of acting always with as much moral integrity as possible, seeking to maximize the patient's autonomy with respect to the mode and conditions of death, knowing that doing so requires that the physician accept and provide information that is discomforting to acknowledge openly. The physician can never wholly dispel anguish but need not despair. Instead of striving always to maximize life, he can pursue the nobler and more arduous task of aiding patients to write as fitting a final chapter as circumstances will allow to the stories of their lives.

10
Progeny, Progress, and Primrose Paths

ISSUES INVOLVING HUMAN SEXUALITY and reproduction are second to none in generating moral debate and in prompting indecision and anxiety. Among the issues that have been highly disputed in one way or another are questions of abortion, birth control, artificial insemination, genetic screening, pornography and censorship, adolescent sexuality, prenatal sex selection, sex-related research and therapy, *in vitro* fertilization, and sex education. Each of these topics has moral dimensions that could fill a volume.

Several of these topics, despite their diversity, share a focus on the status of the human embryo or fetus and the question of what it is permissible to do with one. The mixture of technological progress with sexual matters is also a theme that links a number of topics. In regard to both kinds of issue, individual persons are sometimes faced with difficult moral choices, and there are related questions of public policy, social convention, and law.

I want to look at one aspect of the debate that centers on the use of modern technology as an aid to the fulfillment of the aspirations people have about procreation. In particular, I want to examine the kind of reasoning that the debate inspires because much of it seems to me to be faulty. In this exploration I will focus on issues related to *in vitro* fertilization, but the arguments are plainly of more general relevance.

Not all the moral dilemmas about human sexuality and reproduction are new. Discussion about the morality of abortion goes back for millennia. And selecting the sex of one's children was possible even in ancient times; one simply discarded a newborn baby if the sex was not to one's liking. But modern technology really has changed the dimensions of the debate. For example, it is now possible to identify the sex of a developing fetus by means of amniocentesis, so that parents can abort a fetus if the sex is not what they had hoped for. Obviously people who are opposed to abortion would also be opposed to abortion motivated by a desire to select the sex of one's children. Even some of those who have a moderate position on abortion are uncomfortable about sex selection as a justification. But now the abortion issue may drop out of the debate; recent research on sperm separation techniques suggests that it may become possible to select in advance what the sex of the fetus will be. In that event there will be no question of aborting a fetus of the disappointing sex; parents who want to have a child of a specific sex will arrange for the right kind of insemination. Is that a socially desirable development? Is it right for people to take such a large step in the direction of designing their children to specification, as opposed to welcoming the children, whoever they turn out to be? Opinion is sharply divided on whether the development of the technology to make this prospect a reality would be progress of a beneficial sort or a misuse of scientific knowledge.

The problem of abortion is as socially divisive as any because of the intensity of conviction that disputants bring to it and the apparently ineliminable incompatibility of the various positions they take. At the center of the issue is the status of fetal life. To be explicit, I take the problem to be that of determining the conditions under which it is morally justifiable to perform an abortion, thereby ending the life of a fetus. The two most extreme positions are that abortion is never justified and that it is of no moral consequence. Although each extreme has a few defenders, neither is plausible. Some cases provide such compelling argument in favor of abortion that even most of its opponents reluctantly concede the necessity of terminating the pregnancy. Absolute prohibition has few advocates, even among staunch opponents of abortion. Nor do many deny the moral difficulty of justifying late-stage abortions; the late-stage fetus, after all, is almost indistinguishable from a newborn baby and therefore from a person who, albeit small, is widely believed to have the same sorts of rights and moral standing that larger people have. So most people will agree that the right path lies somewhere between the extremes. But where, and how do we tell?

A parallel dispute exists concerning reproduction by means of *in vitro* fertilization. Wheras abortion is a technique used to end a pregnancy, IVF is a technique used to begin one. Each technique thus plays a role in enabling people to have the sort of family they want; each technique is a part of the growing array of means of controlling our reproductive circumstances.

Many women seek abortions; few need to reproduce by means of IVF. Each technique, however, has become the focus of concern in the forums of public policy. The Supreme Court has made a decision establishing a law of the land in regard to abortion, and federal regulations concerning the use of IVF in clinical and research settings have been debated.

In vitro fertilization is the process by which Louise Brown was conceived. The first of what the journalists call test tube babies, she was born in England in 1978, despite the fact that her mother had an inoperable blockage of the fallopian tubes which prevented her from getting pregnant in the usual way. Physicians removed an egg from Mrs. Brown by means of a surgical procedure, fertilized it in a Petrie dish with sperm from Mr. Brown, nurtured the fertilized egg in the laboratory for several days, then implanted it in Mrs. Brown's uterus. The result was a normal pregnancy and birth. Louise Brown is healthy, famous, and, thanks to a public relations windfall, affluent.

The process used by Drs. Edwards and Steptoe in the case of Louise Brown is complicated, however, by the fact that more than a single egg gets fertilized in the Petrie dish. The technique is just not precise enough to extract and then to fertilize a single egg. (In fact, for the most part, the process doesn't work at all, and it took more than a hundred attempts before the first successful outcome.) So after a fertilized egg is implanted in the womb of the intended mother, the question remains of what to do with the extra eggs that may have been fertilized along the way. The simple answer is to discard them since they are extra, not needed, useless. But two very different objections arise.

To those who believe that personhood begins at conception, the very notion that such entities are valueless and superfluous is distressing. They argue, on the contrary, that the process involves nothing less than callous mass murder of innocent human life, a case of multiple, ex-utero abortion. So the problem of abortion is not merely parallel to the problem of IVF after all but is a part of it.

On the other side are scientists who see great research potential in the use of those extra fertilized eggs as subjects in medical research. If there is anything wrong with discarding the extras, they argue, it is the waste of a valuable opportunity to advance the frontiers of medical knowledge. For if we are concerned to reduce the incidence of congenital illness, there can be no more promising prospect than that of nurturing embryonic life *in vitro*, subjecting it to various environmental influences, and learning thereby how fetal development goes wrong. No event is more tragic than the birth of a grievously defective child; no line of research holds more promise for reducing human tragedy. So the battle lines are drawn.

In the United States there are scientists who want to do research involving IVF and women who want to have children of their own but who, like Mrs. Brown, cannot conceive in the usual way. But there are many who hold that IVF is a procedure that should not be employed—that it is, on moral grounds, a misuse of the physician's art. The government has been in the middle. It provides the funding for most medical research and is thus the target of the scientists' appeals. It is the target of the moral objections as well, and has received 60,000 letters of opposition to the use of IVF.

Let us pursue the debate about *in vitro* fertilization by imagining a woman who desperately wants to have a child of her own, for whom IVF is the only possibility. She is deeply religious, totally committed to doing the morally right thing, aware that there is controversy about the morality of IVF, and unsure what to do. She asks her gynecologist for advice, but the physician is also unsure what to do. She and her colleagues have been asked by a number of patients to make the service available through their practice, either directly or by referral to another clinic. The patient and the physician agree to survey the literature, assess the arguments they find, and try to reach agreement about whether such technologically aided reproduction is an appropriate option. What are the discussions like that they will find?

Laced through the literature of objection to abortion, IVF therapy and research is an argument variously called the primrose path argument, the thin edge of the wedge argument, and the camel's nose in the tent argument. Its structure is familiar: Once one starts sliding down a slippery slope, things get out of control. There is no stopping; disaster awaits us. No skier thinks the argument is generally good; fortunately it is often possible to start down a slippery slope and then to stop.

Paul Ramsey—a prominent Protestant theologian and a leading critic of the use of modern technology in clinical medicine—assures us of disaster in his discussions of such matters, relying heavily, as we shall see, on arguments of this kind. He claims that such measures as artificial insemination and *in vitro* fertilization are the first steps down the primrose path, and there is, in his apocalyptic view, no slowing up, no turning back short of social disaster.[1] Whether or not that view is reasonable is an empirical question. Some processes, like nuclear chain reactions or the spreading of an epidemic, once begun are difficult or impossible to stop. Others are not. It is always an empirical question which sort of process we are dealing with in any particular instance.

I will not attempt to ski the Schilthorn—though I have seen it done—

because my descent, once begun on that insanely precipitous slope, would surely end in cataclysm below. I might as well attempt to ski to safety from a plane in flight. In view of my ability, the argument against my attempting that slope is conclusive. Yet I can handle slopes that beginning skiers properly shun. It is a question of control and judgment.

Is the slippery slope argument against IVF a good one? It is not enough to show that disaster awaits if the process is not controlled. A man walking East in Omaha will drown in the Atlantic—if he does not stop. The argument must also rest on evidence about the likelihood that judgment and control will be exercised responsibly. Here Ramsey's position collapses; he describes disaster and rests his argument on the unduly pessimistic assumption that such unhappy outcomes as are possible will surely occur. But Ramsey sells us short. Collectively we have significant capacity to exercise judgment and control. We have not always done well, especially in areas like foreign policy or energy planning. But our record has been rather good in regard to medical treatment and research.

Consider the vexatious problem of abortion as a case in point. Some opponents of a liberal law have argued that once we allow the killing of fetuses, nothing can stop the slide. If we sanction abortion, they fear, even where amniocentesis reveals a defect like trisomy 21 (Down's Syndrome), we will sanction capricious infanticide as well. If we would abort a fetus on the ground that it is going to be seriously defective, why not allow infanticide on the ground that the child actually has the dreaded defect? Further, such infanticide is just a short skid away from the killing of those judged socially useless, so that if one sanctions early-term abortions even in cases of demonstrable defect, one has irretrievably opened the floodgates to the selective slaughter of anyone in social disfavor.

No such disaster has ensued. Through a process of social policy determination, the society has exercised judgment. That judgment has made a lot of people on both sides unhappy, but it is nonetheless a judgment that makes clear that we can stop a process once we have begun it. Anyone who has ever had a haircut should know that.

Many other examples illustrate our capacity to exercise judgment. Consider an experiment in language acquisition and early child development. We could learn a lot by raising some children in strict isolation from linguistic input for three or four years and then immersing them in a highly verbal environment. No one denies that would be a scientifically sound and useful experiment, but nobody proposes doing it. We will not do so because we judge that on ethical grounds it is indefensible. Andre Hellegers, the late director of the Kennedy Institute for Ethics, and Richard McCormick, a leading Catholic theologian, are right when they speak of "benefits we can never enjoy because we cannot get them without being unethical."[2] There is a difference, despite our mistakes and despite the fears of the pessimists, between what we could do and what we do. That difference is largely due to our capacity for judgment.

Note that with regard to IVF applications, we do not face any single slippery slope argument. Rather, there are several. There are arguments that clinical IVF poses a threat to marriage and the family and to mankind's self-image. There is a separate argument that IVF research will lead to experimentation of an ethically undesirable sort on late-stage fetuses. Each such consideration involves an empirical assessment of the likelihood that sound judgment will prevail as well as an assessment of the magnitude of the disaster if it does not.

It is important here to recognize that the likelihood of the subsequent exercise of judgment and restraint may largely depend on the principles that are used to justify first steps. If early-term abortion were justified by the principle that parents enjoy absolute dominion over their issue, the adoption of that principle would already have constituted a sanctioning of infanticide, and there would be no basis for stopping the slide down the slippery slope. If IVF research on embryos is justified by the principle that prenatal fetal life is of no moral importance, there will be no basis for restraint in regard to research on later-stage fetuses. So it can matter decisively how the justification of first steps is formulated.

There has been considerable speculation about the impact of clinical IVF on marriage and the family. Some of the predictions based on slippery slope arguments are dire. Such prospects as the use of surrogate mothers have been especially disturbing to some writers. (The surrogate mother is a woman who allows the implantation into her uterus of a fertilized egg from another couple, the woman in which wants to have a child of her own but without undergoing pregnancy. The surrogate mother then carries the fetus to term, waiving rights in regard to the resulting child, who is given to the genetic parents.) Hellegers and McCormick warn of such outcomes, toward which they see IVF as leading: "We see in these procedures grave assaults on marriage and the family, to say nothing of the subtle devaluation of sexual intimacy that clings to them."[3] But whereas they raise concerns and call for "a serious public discussion," Ramsey speaks of "what the manipulation of embryos will surely do to ourselves and our progeny."[4] He goes on to invoke the chilling images of a Huxleyan world so sterile that "there is no poetry."[5]

These issues are of the first importance. But it is necessary not to lose sight, in the glare of that importance, of the need to examine the evidence. What reason is there to give credence to such portents of familial disaster?

Much of the case seems based on concern about the separation of reproduction from sexual intercourse. But artifical insemination, with husbands' and with donors' sperm, has been practiced widely, if not very visibly, for decades. There has been no discernible deleterious effect on marriage or the family. More important, the wide availability of inexpensive and effective birth control means that for the first time in human history, sex and reproduction have already been separated. The impact on social structure will surely be astounding; no doubt it will transcend our current understanding. So it is a wholly idle worry that IVF will separate sex and procreation.

It is worth remembering, moreover, that IVF involves hospitalization and surgery, and it is a very small percentage of the population that is in any position to benefit from it. The traditional method of conception will remain the method of choice. It is inexpensive, can be performed at home, takes little time, training, or skill, and is a great deal of fun. I do not see it in serious jeopardy.

Further, we are only beginning to document what we have known all along: that there is no substitute for early parent-child interaction.[6] As we learn more fully how the family works when it is working well, I suspect that our appreciation of it and of its special capacity for nurturing will grow. Hellegers and McCormick are right; we should take the long view and look at societal consequences, not simply at individual needs, in evaluating IVF. But I do not see the family under grave assault because of IVF. Indeed, it is often a respect for family, lineage, and the traditional parental role that prompts the request for clinical IVF in the first place.

Finally, mankind's image of what it is to be human may well involve a sense of lineage and of parenting, and that image may undergo some perturbation from the few cases in which procreation has a heavy dose of technology added. But mankind's sense of what it is to be human is threatened far more seriously on other fronts. Recent work on primate language acquisition, notwithstanding debate about its significance, has challenged the belief that we alone have the capacity for abstraction or to communicate to others a sense of self-awareness, and in the process the sharpness of the distinction between humans and the higher primates has been blunted.[7] Recent work in artificial intelligence has produced machines with awesome cognitive capacities, and the sharpness of the distinction between people and machines has also been challenged.[8] We have ample reason to reflect seriously about what we are. The prospects for IVF add little to the case.

Like the slippery slope argument, the concept of what is natural plays a frequent role in the writings of those who are troubled by IVF. Ramsey, for example, writes:

> Today many are testifying to the spiritual autonomy of all natural objects and to arrogance over none; to the scheme of things in which man has his place. But there is as yet no discernible evidence that we are recovering a sense for man as a natural object, too, toward whom a like form of "natural piety" is appropriate. . . . [P]rocreation, parenthood, is certainly one of those "courses of action" natural to man, which cannot without violation be disassembled and put together again—any more than we have the wisdom or the right impiously to destroy the environment of which we are a part rather than working according to its lineaments, according to the functions we discover to be the case in the whole assemblage of natural objects.[9]

He then goes on to advocate the position that "the proper objective of medicine is to serve and care for man as a natural object, to help in all our natural 'courses of action,' to tend the garden of our creation."[10] It is time this sort of argument was laid permanently to rest. That something is natural has, by itself, absolutely no moral force.

We can distinguish three senses in which an action or process can be said to be natural:

1. It conforms to the laws of nature; the contrast, I presume, is with the impossible or with the supernatural. But *everything* we do or could do—the good and bad alike—is natural in this sense. No moral distinctions can be based on it.

2. It is free of human intervention; the contrast is with processes influenced by mankind's efforts to manipulate its environment. But *nothing* we do is natural in this sense, for our action is itself the mark of the unnatural. The practice of medicine itself is a clear example of human efforts to manipulate the playing out of events, as when we deliberately destroy "natural" life forms and terminate a "natural" process by using antibiotics to cure an infection. No moral distinctions can be based on this sense of what is natural either.

3. It conforms to some natural moral law or other code or set or principles of value; the contrast here is with what is wrong, what is a violation of principles about how one ought to act. In this interpretation the concept of what is natural has moral force, but only because it is based on some prior judgment about what is right and what is wrong— a judgment then reflected in the choice of what to call natural and artificial.

The passage from Ramsey suggests that he employs the third sense of *natural*; that he sees certain processes, such as normal procreation, as desirable; and that he extols their naturalness without thereby suggesting that medical intervention is typically a violation of nature.

The claim of naturalness is thus a moral *conclusion*, not evidence that can be offered in a moral argument. Ramsey sees atypical reproduction as undesirable but says little about why. His invocation of the concept of the natural only obscures the point that there are morally desirable and morally undesirable actions, and we must strive to discern the difference between them on reasonable grounds, not on purported grounds of naturalness. I do not understand why this confusion about the moral significance of the concept of what is natural persists as widely and tenaciously as it does.

The most central issue in the debate about IVF, however, as in the debate about abortion, is the question of the status of the embryo. In approaching this question, we must recall the crucial distinction between facts we seek to discover and decisions we need to make. If we wish to know a fact, we seek to discover it through appropriate research. Contrast that with the question of when a young person becomes an adult. Whether a person warrants classification as an adult at thirteen, eighteen, or twenty-one is not a fact to discover through research in biology, physiology, psychology, or anything else. It is social policy, a decision of the body politic. This distinction between discoveries and decisions seems straightforward, yet sometimes the two become confused. Much discussion about death, for example, proceeds on the misconception that the criterion of death is a fact to discover. Yet as we saw in the last chapter, the appropriate criterion of death in clinical situations is not a fact to discover; it is a social policy to make. (That is one reason why the results of such discussions are somewhat unstable, why the criterion of death is a subject of ongoing dispute; the factors that go into justifying a social policy decision are always open to review and to argument.)

What, then, of the embryo—the embryo that is implanted and the embryo that is dealt with otherwise? Inevitably there arise questions of whether or not such embryos are persons or are the bearers of rights. These are not questions of fact but instead require the setting of social policy. To say that a question is a question of policy is not to say that the answers are unconstrained. There are clear cases of life and of death; the question arises—and a policy is needed—only in cases at the margin where some physiological systems still function while others are irretrievably lost. So the range within which decision can be made is rather narrow. Similarly, the questions of what to count as a person and what to count as a bearer of rights require decision only within a circumscribed range—the cases at the margins of personhood. Such cases are of various sorts—the anencephalic newborn, the linguistically proficient primate, the embryo.

I will not rehearse the extensive debate about the personhood of embryos and fetuses, a debate fueled by intense division of sentiment about abortion. Rather, I will sketch the conclusions that seem to me to provide the most reasonable basis for judgment.

Surely the concept of a person involves in some fundamental way the capacity for sentience, for an awareness of sensations at the very least. In the normal case there is much more. There is self-awareness, capacity for reflection, a sense of others and of relationships between self and others. So the condition of sentience is very weak, a necessary condition for personhood, but far from a sufficient condition.

No one seriously contends that embryos are sentient, that they are capable of even the slightest awareness of pleasure or pain. Of course, if all goes well, they will develop into people, and it is on that potential that the case for their personhood largely rests. The idea of potential is tricky. We often hear encomiums to it: Individuals should have the opportunity to fulfill their potential, it is somehow grounds for disappointment when someone fails to live up to his potential, and the like. But that is careless talk, for some potentials are desirable and others are not. He who has the potential to be Sherlock Holmes has the potential to be a master criminal; she who has the manual dexterity for neurosurgery perhaps has the potential to be a leading pickpocket as well. Further, he who has the potential to be a swimmer and to be a ballet dancer must choose between them; what advances one potential interferes with the other. So aphorisms about potential do little to advance the debate. Mainly what they come to is that it is good to advance those potentials that it is good to advance.

Even though *people* should be encouraged in living up to some of their more desirable potentials, we cannot use that principle to defend a claim that *embryos* have personhood or rights since the principle is about the potentials of persons—and whether or not embryos should be accorded that status is precisely the point in question. It is not obvious that rights should accrue to an object just because it has the potential, assuming that all goes well, to become a person at some later time. Indeed, the unfertilized human egg, like the embryo, has the potential to become a person if all goes well—when all going well includes getting fertilized. And no one has argued that each unfertilized egg or each spermatozoon be accorded personhood or rights.

One does hear it said of the embryo that it has the potential to become a *particular* adult person. Its genetic identity is complete; it is already a unique individual. That does distinguish it from spermatozoa and ova in isolation (apart from the possibility of twinning), but not from identified, though unjoined, pairs of sperm and egg. That no union has yet occurred does not alter the fact that any pair of sperm and egg has the potential, if all goes well, to become a genetically specific adult person. The point of conception may be, for some, a convenient place to draw the line, but there should be no mistake about the fact that it is drawn there for convenience. That is no less "arbitrary" a choice than the choice to draw the line later, which I believe it makes better sense to do. Indeed, it is a myth that conception is itself instantaneous. Even one who seeks to avoid the problem of "drawing a line" by choosing conception as an unproblematic point is in reality selecting a temporal region within which a process takes place over time. That we did not know this fact before it was possible to monitor the process of conception at the microscopic level does not make it any the less important a fact.

At the other end of fetal development we are struck by the similarity between infants and late-stage fetuses. Indeed, not only is the late-stage fetus clearly sentient, reacting to stimuli in its environment, but in most cases it already holds a place, as a specific, though unseen, individual, in a network of human emotions and expectations. In most respects it is like a child and utterly unlike an embryo.

For my part, the onset of the capacity for sentience marks a qualitative change in fetal development. From that point forward what we do may cause it, as a present actuality, to suffer. Surely that is a morally significant factor, though not the only one. It is an empirical question of neurological development when that change occurs; it happens sometime prior to quickening but well after the embryonic stage. That we have no word for this stage in the series of events that includes conception, quickening, and birth reflects only the fact that we have not historically invested it with much significance or until recently had much understanding of the development of which it is a part. It is not necessarily less significant for that.

The later it is in its development, the more seriously we should take a fetus as a person in the making. I see no reason for, and no possibility of, holding to a clear-cut distinction between the nonperson and the person as if personhood somehow snaps into place in an instant, instead of emerging organically out of a developmental process. That emergence, I suggest, begins to have moral force with the onset of fetal sentience. In any case, I know of no persuasive arguments for the position that the most reasonable social policy is to accord the embryo the status of a person.

Leon Kass, a physician and persuasive commentator on ethical issues in medicine, has argued forcefully that the human embryo is an entity of moral significance:

The human blastocyst, even the blastocyst *in vitro*, is not humanly nothing; it possesses a power to become what everyone will agree is a human being. . . . [T]he blastocyst is not nothing, it is *at least* potential humanity, and as such it elicits, or ought to elicit, our feelings of awe and respect. In the blastocyst, even in the zygote, we face a mysterious and awesome power. . . . *The human embryo is not mere meat; it is not just stuff; it is not a thing.* Because of its origin and because of its capacity, it commands a higher respect.[11]

I agree that the human blastocyst is not humanly nothing. So, too, however, do all the advocates of IVF. It is *precisely* the human blastocyst's potential to become a human being that makes it an object of particular research interest and that accounts for the possibility of clinical IVF. From the fact that it is not humanly nothing, no conclusion directly follows about what should or should not be done.

Of course, the force of Kass's argument is intended to rest not merely on the fact that the human blastocyst has some human status but on its mysterious and awesome power, its capacity to engender awe and respect. But it is not the *human* character of the blastocyst that accounts for its splendor. Any strand of DNA confronts us with a mysterious and awesome power; any mammalian embryo embodies an "immanent plan" that dwarfs our understanding; any acorn is, as much as anything ever is, miraculous; and even the lowly hydrogen atom, reflected on with reverent disposition, is humbling in its beauty, power, and complexity. And so are cathedrals, symphonies, great literary works, and the minds of great scientists.

Surely, one might claim, I miss the point. Human blastocysts are not uniquely grounds for awe, but they do command, as Kass puts it, a "higher respect." He is not explicit, however, in the comparison; higher than what, one wonders. The context suggests an answer: higher than the respect commanded by "mere meat," by that which is "just stuff." But two problems of interpreting the point arise. First, Kass nowhere explains what he means by *respect*. He has merely *invoked* the notion of the respect due the embryo, much as Ramsey invoked the notion of the natural. Secondly, Kass does not consider the respect due to other objects than the embryo. That omission is what gives plausibility to his argument that since human blastocysts are due respect, they ought not be the subjects of research or clinical manipulation. Kass, I am certain, would agree that human cadavers should be treated with respect; they are not mere meat, not humanly nothing, not unrelated to a network of emotional attachments and deeply felt values that constrain how we treat the bodily remains of former persons. Yet Kass does not protest the use of cadavers in medical education or the practice of transplanting organs from someone who has just died. To be sure, there is a difference between using cadavers and abusing them, and it is to this difference that the concept of respect is relevant. It is simply a mistake to assume that if an object is due respect, it is therefore wrong to make practical use of it.

Finally, Kass speaks freely of the appropriateness of experimenting on animals, including primates. But are animals not also due respect? They are sentient creatures whose development and behavior are proper grounds for awe and wonder, they participate in social communities, and in some cases their communicative capacity is far greater than we had until recently imagined. The homocentricity of Kass's position enables him to make respect sound like a barrier to use. In fact, it is a barrier only to abuse. If we can justifiably experiment on animals under some circumstances, and if we can justifiably make use of human remains, despite the fact that they are not humanly nothing, I see no reason based on the concept of respect why we cannot, respectfully, make justifiable clinical and research use of human blastocysts.

Both Kass and R. G. Edwards, in reply to Kass, have discussed the proper function of medicine and whether IVF is defensible in terms of it. There are serious issues here. Kass argues:

> Just as infertility is not a disease, so providing a child by artificial means to a woman with blocked oviducts is not treatment. . . . What is being "treated" is her desire—a perfectly normal and unobjectional desire—to bear a child.[12]

Ramsey voices a similar concern:

> The important line lies between doctoring desires . . . and seeking to correct a medical condition if it is possible to do so. . . . [M]edical practice loses its way into an entirely different human activity—manufacture . . . if it undertakes either to produce a child without curing infertility as a condition or to produce simply the desired sort of child.[13]

Edwards replies:

> A great many medical advances depend on the replacement of a deficient compound or an organ. Examples include insulin, false teeth, and spectacles: the clinical condition itself remains, but treatment modifies its expression. Patients taking advantage of these three treatments are surely receiving the correct therapeutic measures, the doctors treating the desire to be nondiabetic or to see and eat properly. . . . Exactly the same argument applies to the cure of infertility:

should patients have their desired children, the treatment would have achieved its purpose.[14]

We need not rely on the idea of prosthetic devices to make Edwards's point that treatment does often leave the initial condition unaltered while responding to a patient's desire to transcend the limitations imposed by that condition. The administration of tranquilizers, sleeping pills, and analgesics are examples of medical treatments which do not correct physiological deficiencies but respond, in a sense, to a patient's desires. Edwards's defense seems adequate; treating some desires is a traditional and appropriate part of medical practice.

But the problem runs deeper, for it may not be appropriate to treat all medically treatable desires. First, there is the question of the distribution of costs, a question that has heightened impact if we consider the use of public funds to pay for medical treatment. It is one thing to provide insulin, dialysis, or dentures to a patient. But should we provide cosmetic surgery when the desire does not arise out of injury or illness but rather is simply a wish to be more youthfully attractive? Perhaps such treatment is unexceptionable if the costs are borne wholly by the patient. But other desires arising out of vanity seem less legitimate. Should surgical treatment have been available to those women who, in the 1950s, had their little toes amputated in order to fit their feet into narrower and hence, in their benighted judgment, more fashionable shoes? Or is the provision of such treatment a misuse of medical skills, a perversion of the privilege that the license to practice medicine signifies? I submit that this is the case and that the underlying reason is that the treatment of a desire for self-mutilation in the service of a whimsical vanity is not the sort of desire that legitimately warrants treatment.

As we saw in chapter 6, value-free medicine is not fully possible. Some judgments about which desires are properly treatable, and which not, must be made. We cannot oppose clinical IVF on the ground that it is the treatment of a desire, nor can we simply approve it on the ground, as Edwards suggests, that the treatment of desires is medically legitimate. Rather, we must face directly the question of whether the desire to have a child of one's own, when IVF is the only available means, is one of the desires that warrants medical response.

At this point our hypothetical patient and physician, if they agree with me, will conclude that there is no adequate argument against the clinical use of IVF as a response to inoperable infertility. But they may remain troubled by some of the dangers to which critics like Ramsey, Hellegers, McCormick, and Kass call our attention, despite the weaknesses in their arguments. For there remains something discomforting about the notion of raising embryos in the laboratory for use as research subjects, notwithstanding the useful knowledge that might result. And there remains something discomforting about the growing incidence of surrogate motherhood arrangements that have already begun to lead us into uncharted waters of litigation, as when the surrogate mother decides during the pregnancy to try to keep the child she had agreed to incubate for someone else. But these problems must be faced on their own, and the judgments we make in response to them should remain distinguishable from the judgments we make about more straightforward uses of IVF as a clinical therapy. We need not consider all possible uses of IVF as parts of one inseparable package any more than we need endorse an absolutist position on abortion. There is no good reason why we cannot separate justifiable from unjustifiable instances on the basis of where the best arguments lie.

We have considered a number of issues relating to clinical decisions that raise questions of public policy. Abortion is a paradigm case since there is ongoing public debate about how the law should limit the range within which clinical and personal judgments are made. Many other aspects of clinical medicine are touched by the outcome of public policy debates regarding the legal definition of death, the collection and allocation of transplantable organs, the use of public funds to underwrite the costs of medical services, and the like. It is time we considered the question of how public policy should be determined in respect to such morally disputed matters.*

*Philosophers over the last decade have come to play an increasingly active role as participants in the analysis and formulation of public policy. From 1975 to 1979, for example, twenty-five different federal agencies hired philosophers as consultants.[15] In keeping with this trend, in October of 1978 I was asked by the Ethics Advisory Board of the Department of Health, Education, and Welfare (now Health and Human Services) to testify on the moral permissibility of *in vitro* fertilization. Much of this chapter is based on the testimony I presented.

In June of 1979, the Secretary of Health, Education, and Welfare published a notice in the *Federal Register* including the recommendations of the Board concerning the ethical acceptability of research involving IVF. No action has been taken on these recommendations. At this writing (November 1981), such research is still prohibited under a federal moratorium, and a proposal requesting support for such research is still pending, having been submitted in 1977 and approved on its scientific merits before being referred to the Board for consideration of the ethical issues. The debate that preceded the Board's recommendations on IVF, like the earlier deliberations of the National Commission for the Protection of Human Subjects of Biomedical Research and the subsequent discussions of the President's Commission for the Study of Ethical Problems in Medicine and Biomedical and Behavioral Research (appointed by President Carter in August 1979), was marked by the involvement of lawyers, clergymen, members of the public, philosophers, and many others from outside the scientific and medical communities. Public hearings were held in every region of the country. Such inquiries can be expected to increase as the public takes an increasingly active interest in the ethical dimensions of scientific and medical activities; it should be useful, therefore, to bear in mind some of the concepts, issues, arguments, and principles that shape the results of such debates.

11
Setting Public Policy

THE ISSUES IN CLINICAL MEDICINE that I have discussed thus far pertain primarily to the making of choices by individual patients and health care providers. Such choices are always made within such larger contexts as the hospital, with its rules and standard procedures; the medical specialty, with its conventions of practice; the patient's religious tradition, with its positions on matters of morality; the social community, with its mechanisms of approval and disapproval; the law, with its various sanctions; and others. Sometimes the decision faced by an individual is not restrained by these larger contexts, as when a patient must choose either continued medical management of moderate angina pectoris or coronary arterial bypass surgery. In other situations the larger context impinges directly on the possibilities of choice. If abortion were outlawed again, a woman seeking an abortion would have to choose among going to an illegal abortionist, traveling to another country, or continuing the pregnancy. And if the law requires that newly minted physicians spend a year or two in underserved parts of the country, the range of choices about the early years of practice will be sharply limited. So questions of policy regarding medical matters can be distinguished from questions of clinical decision and individual choice, but the two levels of concern do interact.

This chapter represents something of a departure from the main themes of our discussion. I will focus here on a few of the issues that arise when we shift our attention from individual choice to the arenas of public policy. That shift was implicit in the discussion of *in vitro* fertilization, where the arguments pertained both to what our hypothetical patient and physician should do and to what sorts of policies should be adopted by clinics, insurers, public health agencies, and the law. I will return to the question of how public policy should be set regarding matters that are morally charged and vigorously disputed, but first I want to explore some of the concepts that arise especially in discussions of policy.

Such discussions often center on questions related to scarcity and cost. Although the allocation of scarce resources is commonly addressed at the level of policy, the result can determine what transactions can take place between physician and patient. Among the scarce goods I have in mind are physicians willing to work in poor or rural areas, dollars to pay for costly medical technology, newly developed drugs or devices that are not yet in plentiful supply, and transplantable tissue, such as corneas or kidneys. Not only are the costs associated with the supply and distribution of such goods monetary, but they also involve considerations of individual freedom and of health, as when physicians are reassigned to locations they did not choose or when a person donates a kidney to save a sibling.

In the attempt to establish policies to deal with any of these issues, we commonly express the desire to obtain and distribute health care resources in a way that is both efficient and equitable. But we are not adequately clear about what efficiency and equity are. I will illustrate by examining the problem of providing an adequate supply of live organs for kidney transplantation.

When we speak of efficiency, we tend to do so in a way that reflects the usage of that notion in physics or engineering. There efficiency is a calculable ratio—the ratio of work output to work input—which approaches the value one as a limiting and unachievable ideal. Every machine has an efficiency, every efficiency is a number, and any two efficiencies can therefore be compared. But when we leave the realm of physics, we leave its precision behind. Our talk of efficiency in other contexts suffers from the tempting but false assumption that it is still a precise notion, quite serviceable for making quantitative decisions. The vagueness is not eliminated merely by dressing the old notion of efficiency in the fancy new clothes of cost-benefit or cost-effectiveness language.

Consider two automobile engines mounted on a bench. Engine A, which can propel a two-ton car for twenty-five miles on a gallon of gasoline, hums smoothly on the bench. Engine B can propel a two-ton car for only fifteen miles on a gallon of the same gasoline at the same speed. It sits on the bench, clattering and sputtering, whistling and clanging. Which is the more efficient engine? So long as propelling cars is at issue, of course, Engine A is more efficient. But if I am a movie producer at work on the sound track of a film about antique automobiles, and what I am after is the most automotive engine clatter I can get per gallon, then obviously Engine B is more efficient.

Implicit in any use of the notion of efficiency is an assumption about what the desired outcome is. In classical physics, it is well defined. In ordinary discourse about cars, it is contextually implied. In the example of the two engines, it was hidden at first and perhaps surprising when revealed.

When we talk about efficiency in health care, what exactly are the values and the output products in terms of which—and only in terms of which—we can make sense of claims about efficiency? We have not answered this question in any adequate way. But until we reach clarity about what the output objectives of medical care are to be, we cannot usefully make more than impressionistic judgments about efficiency.

If a large investment by a hospital in a hyperbaric chamber enables it to save a few lives each year, is that an efficient investment compared with supporting a community diagnostic program that could improve the health of thousands of people? Is a multimillion dollar public immunization program an efficient investment of health care dollars if it protects most of the population at risk against an epidemic of unknown likelihood? These questions are not merely hard to answer. Rather, the questions themselves are unclear. They use a notion of efficiency which is not well defined or well understood.

We often spend a great deal to save the life of an identified person. We are less likely to invest in the statistical saving of lives—to incur expenses that will save the lives of persons unspecified, for example, by building bridges over all railroad crossings. Sometimes, however, we invest heavily to that end—for instance, in the establishment of a shock-trauma unit. Yet we do not make all the investments that would surely save lives, in part because we are not sure how important to us it is to save all the lives it is medically possible to save. Further, it is impossible to compare such an investment with one that provides nonvital medical care without understanding what value we place on good health. It is not obvious, anyway, that we clearly favor saving a few lives over substantially improving the well-being of a large number of people.

These questions, of course, are not for philosophy to answer alone. They are problems of social decision, and the answers should be fashioned by all those whose risk and whose resources are involved. Moreover, the question of what to take as the appropriate objective in terms of which to evaluate efficiency itself depends on considerations of equity.

Turn, then, to equity—what common usage and the dictionary both take as equivalent to justice, fairness, doing the right thing. There are various competing views of what constitutes equity. One prominent view is that equity is or requires *equality*. What might that mean in the context of the distribution of health care? There are at least these choices:

1. Equality in the dollar expenditure on each individual. This interpretation makes little sense. Some lucky people just don't need health care; they thrive until they die, and there isn't anything to spend their health care dollars on. Perhaps we could approximate an equal expenditure by allocating to each person some fixed amount—say, $100,000—over his lifetime, with a refund of any unused portion to go to his estate.

2. Equality in the state of health of each individual. The problem here is that this sort of equality is impossible no matter what we spend or how. Some people enjoy robust health, some are sickly or worse all their lives, and we have only limited leverage on the natural distribution of physiological characteristics.

3. Equality in the maximum to which each individual is benefited. This would mean that each person has equal access to medical care up to some limit, to be drawn on as needed, with no pretense of equalizing actual expenditures. We may find this becoming a position to be taken seriously, though the question of what sorts of limits should be set is just beginning to rear its vexatious head.

4. Equality in the treatment of like cases. Under this interpretation, a national health service, for example, could have a program in renal dialysis, treating as needed all medically qualified cases. At the same time it could refuse to treat cases of hemophilia at all, arguing that such an exclusion was necessary on grounds of economy and going on to claim that the health care was wholly equitable, thoroughly equal, in the sense that each person had equal claim on such treatments as were made available. Both the patient with kidney failure and the hemophiliac would have equal access to dialysis as needed according to this plan.

So if we interpret equity as equality in some sense or other, we immediately face problems of interpretation. Each interpretation, moreover, is problematic. It is not clear or unchallenged that any sort of egalitarian interpretation of equity is tenable. First, there will always be some medical treatments or materials in short supply—at least the ones that have just been developed. How are we to achieve equality here except by a lottery that provides not equal treatment, but an equal *chance* of getting treatment? Secondly, there is the problem of entitlement. Consider the research scientist who has devoted his life to the search for a vaccine for a disease that has slaughtered his ancestors for generations. Now he has the vaccine, but initially in short supply. Are we to deny his claim on a dose for himself or his child because that would violate equal access? Many would argue that he has an entitlement that sets him apart from the rest; that to deny it would itself to be to abandon our commitment to equity.

So equity, like efficiency—although for different reasons—is an elusive notion. We rely on them both in the rhetoric that surrounds the defense of policy, and we rely on our intuitions about them in the setting and advocacy of policy. But when it comes to a specific case of defending a policy under careful scrutiny, these notions slip away from precise clarification. What, then, is to be said for them?

One way to interpret the notion of efficiency—a way that seems to correspond well with the way we actually use it—is as a measure of the extent to which an action produces good—where *good* is itself defined as the satisfaction of human needs and desires. That action, program, or policy then is most efficient which, at a given level of expenditure, maximizes good. Comparative judgments are then possible to the degree to which we are clear about what is good and also about what consequences will flow from the various acts we contemplate.

This is classical utilitarianism, the influence of which has dominated not only moral philosophy for the last century but economics and Anglo-American legislative policy as well. The objections to it, as we have seen, are numerous and powerful, but its appeal nonetheless remains strong as an account of what we ought to do, individually and collectively, and why. This appeal rests ultimately on the simple fact that we do care about the satisfaction of human wants and needs—about the production of good—and we therefore want our efforts and our resources to produce as much of it as possible. This want translates into our concern with efficiency.

Equity is a more obviously moral notion. It means justice, fairness in our dealings with one another. But how are we to understand what is just? From the ancient Pythagorean rules of conduct and the Ten Commandments through the austere moral strictures of Kant to an extensive body of anti-utilitarian moral theory, we have sustained the sense that some kinds of actions are right and other kinds are wrong, regardless of the consequences they lead to or the ends they serve, simply because of the kinds of acts they are. Thus, we condemn the framing of an innocent man, no matter how great the social benefits of the conviction might be, just as we condemn torture, slavery, and other moral abominations without regard to the role they may play in the larger pursuit of noble ends.

Mill's view that justice is derivative from considerations of utility, of efficiency in the production of good results, is in decline. Recent moral philosophy has shown reluctance to consider justice as a derivative concept. Rather, it has come to be largely viewed as a dimension of morality that is separate from and independent of utility and that can therefore be in conflict with it.

Efficiency as a value thus reflects our concern with the maximum production of good, and equity as a value reflects our concern with doing what is just or fair, regardless of its efficiency. In an ideal world these values would never be in conflict, but in fact the conflict is notorious. We may want both equity and efficiency, but at least sometimes one may be purchased only at the cost of the other.

To see the conflict between equity and efficiency etched sharply, consider a hypothetical example similar to that which introduced Rawls's views about justice. (The complexity of real cases can too easily obscure even a simple point.) Imagine that we all are on a desert island, struggling to survive. Most of us cluster into a village, but a few set out for remote parts of the island, where the fishing is perhaps better. There is little rain, so drinking water is a constant problem; there is just marginally enough to keep us alive. Suddenly a rescue mission flies overhead. Using remote sensing technology, they assess our situation. They depart, then return with a large crate which they parachute to the island. We open the crate and find a tank truck filled with pure water and a message that the water is for all the people on the island. How shall we distribute the water?

There are 100 people on the island; 1,000 gallons in the tank. Specify whatever distribution you think equitable. You can favor 10 gallons per person, or more for those who work more, or most for those in positions of authority—it doesn't matter which distribution you favor as most equitable. For you now discover that the tank truck has a steam engine. In order to move it around at all, you have to use water. And the conflict between efficiency and equity—however you construe equity—becomes plain. Assuming that each gallon of water is as valuable to each person as any other gallon (that is, there is no diminishing marginal utility of water in the range of quantities at issue), the most efficient thing to do is not to use the engine at all. Let water go to those who come for it— to the able-bodied who live nearby. The weak, the ill, the aged, the distant will get none. Since there is linearity in the good produced by incremental allocations of water, their deprivation is of no consequence, for we produce more good this way than by wasting some of the water on operating the delivery truck. It would be hard to argue that justice is served, however, especially in view of the fact that the water was sent to all the people on the island.

So equity costs something. In some situations the most efficient action and the most equitable action are not the same. Some balance must then be struck between the two competing values. For one who places justice above all, considerations of efficiency may legitimately come into play, but only after justice is fully served. This position would be exemplified by the egalitarian who insisted on an equal distribution of water to all island inhabitants even if most of the water were used by delivering it. But he could still be seriously concerned with mapping the best route, in order to conserve water, and thus to distribute it most efficiently within the constraints of equity. He would be the mirror image of the complete utilitarian who advocated making the decision solely on grounds of efficiency and therefore leaving the truck in place. For many people, myself among them, some middle ground is best—some approximation to complete equity, tempered by an unwillingness to let efficiency fall too low.

I have not shown, of course, that equity and efficiency are always in conflict—only that they are competing values in some situations. It is a separate question whether the situations in health care are of the sort in which equity and efficiency are in conflict. But the conflict is clearly present. In the early days of renal dialysis we had a classic problem of allocating limited vital resources. There were not enough machines to go around. That problem is now essentially past, but a similar situation exists with respect to live-organ transplants. Many more patients are medically qualified to receive transplanted kidneys than can be accommodated under the present rate of supply. How shall we respond to this situation?

Various principles of distribution come to mind. Consider:

1. To each according to his means. This is a free-market policy. Kidneys go to those who can afford them, with the price determined by market phenomena.

2. To each according to his social utility. This is roughly the approach adopted in the original dialysis selection in Seattle, where an assessment was made of the social utility of the applicants. It is the utilitarian approach, the one that seeks to maximize efficiency.

3. To each according to his entitlement or status. A policy like this might favor veterans, landowners, members of the party in power, or other groups or individuals making special claims.

4. To each according to his luck. This is the policy of the strict egalitarian: Count every medically qualified individual as an equal, and draw lots to determine who will get the kidneys.

5. To each according to his need. To implement this policy, of course, requires an increase in the supply of the resource the scarcity of which presents the problem in the first place.

The choice among these distributional policies will be difficult because our values do not all point to a single choice. In particular, we are sympathetic both to considerations of social utility and to the desirability of meeting everyone's need where we have the ability to meet anyone's. So there is a pressure to increase service to meet demand, thereby to eliminate some of the conflict we feel, and that yields pressure to increase the supply of transplantable kidneys while keeping a lid on the costs. Is there any possibility of doing that?

ABC News reported in the Autumn of 1978 that recent legislation in France makes a person's organs available at death for transplantation unless the individual has exercised a prior option of objection. Should we adopt a similar policy? The government could go a step beyond France, requiring organ donation without option of prior objection. Or it could go two steps beyond, drafting people into a national organ bank battalion. These people might be selected if they are in good health, late in life, and of low social utility. They would then be required to donate one kidney, with the rest of their organs to be taken at death. The French policy is moderate in the context of what is possible. Still, it is seen as overly coercive by many critics. Milder measures include a proposal made by an officer of the American Kidney Foundation, who suggested that each individual agree or decline at the time of registration with the Social Security Administration. But Sidney Wolfe, of the Health Research Group, responded that any such association with a government agency that provides vital support services could be implicitly coercive. Still milder measures are available, however. The government could decide to support the present system of total voluntarism with a campaign aimed at persuading large numbers of people to become donors. Or the government could leave the matter wholly to the workings of the private sector.

For an illuminating comparison, consider briefly a different problem. We provide military manpower in various ways at various times depending not only on our national security needs but also on our moral priorities. The draft, favored in wartime, is the most efficient way to provide the manpower, especially combined with selective deferment. The government conscripts soldiers, paying what it decides to pay—thereby containing payroll costs—and exempting those whose greater social utility lies elsewhere—thereby maximizing social efficiency. The principle is: from each according to his usefulness. But this policy is criticized on grounds of equity. It sends the poor and underprivileged off to battle, favoring further the already favored, while the benefit of national defense—that is, the security of the nation—is equally enjoyed by all. Moved by conscience to provide military manpower more equitably, we change to a lottery.

Now the principle is: from each according to his luck in an equal-risk lottery. But this policy has critics, for it obliterates the freedom of the unlucky draftee and reduces efficiency by drafting some who would be more usefully placed elsewhere. So out of respect for personal liberty we move to a volunteer service: from each according to his choice. Freedom is honored, but the costs soar because the incentive to join is not great for most people in a reasonably sound economy. And now we hear lamentation from the Pentagon: We have liberty; but the price is getting beyond our reach, and the efficiency is low. So once again we may move to another system, striking a different balance among the competing values of efficiency, equality, and liberty.

A parallel situation exists in regard to kidney supply and distribution. The various plans clearly exhibit different degrees of respect for different values. A plausible utilitarian case can be made for the very coercive plans to increase supply, and as we move through the shadings of coercion from a draft or universal requirement, to coercion of varying degrees, to persuasion, education, and voluntarism, the level of efficiency seems to drop. At the same time the level of equity in the treatment of persons seems to rise, especially if we take equity to require respect for personal autonomy and the bodily integrity of individual persons. But now a curious bind seems to emerge. For if the most equitable policy for distribution requires meeting the needs of all patients who require transplants, that policy also seems to require, as a practical matter, a highly efficient policy for obtaining transplantable kidneys. Yet the policies that seem most efficient in this regard seem least equitable from the point of view of potential donors. Thus, we see equity not only in opposition to efficiency but to equity itself.

A second example reinforces the point. Assume that considerations of equity—of justice or fairness in the treatment of persons—require that each individual be free to choose the geographical location in which he or she will seek work. Assume further that considerations of equity require that in an affluent industrialized nation like ours a minimally decent level of health care should be available to all citizens, including those in poor, rural communities. Finally, assume that our concern with containing the costs of health care places limits on the amount of financial incentive we can provide to induce physicians to practice in otherwise undesirable locations. Then the conflict is evident: We can resolve the problem only by some sacrifice in the freedom of the physician, the health care of the poor, or the pocketbook of the public. And any such sacrifice will be to some extent a concession with respect to either equity or efficiency.

We need, in our deliberations about health policy, a more sophisticated understanding of how to assess the costs and the values of the various outcomes that health care provides. Slogans about efficiency or equity will do us no more good than those about potential or the natural. My own view is that we tend to weigh efficiency too heavily in its conflict with equity in part because of the difficulty of measuring the value of considerations of equity. Perhaps the basic mistake is to assume that what is needed is *measurement* at all, as opposed to the informed and sensitive judgment that lies at the heart of leadership and statesmanship.

One final example: Imagine a large family next door. They treat all their children well except the youngest. That one is neglected, disdained— an outcast. We would, I think, judge that family harshly, accepting as a mark of its degree of decency the way it treats the one whom it treats least well. Similarly, the keystone of Rawls's theory of justice is respect for liberty conjoined with concern for the least advantaged among us. Those who suffer from debilitating illness or handicap are, in an important sense, the least advantaged among us, and we neglect them at our own moral risk. There is no way to assign a dollar value to such considerations, and they may in tragic circumstances even be defeasible on grounds of excessive cost. Nonetheless, they have a force that should not be under-estimated.

It may be useful to keep Rawls's criterion in mind as a *prima facie* constraint on our pursuit of efficiency. That constraint would prevent us from assessing health care policies in a purely utilitarian way or in a way that excludes the interests of any segment of the population. It would not by itself determine what policies we should set, but by narrowing the range of choices, it would play some role in the process. Setting public policies for health care that are equitable and affordable is always a complex task, and it would be futile to expect any stable resolution of policy to be achieved. Rather, there must be an ongoing process of assessment and reassessment in the public and political forums.

Some policies, of course, are set at relatively local levels. A Catholic hospital, for example, may reasonably prohibit abortion within its walls, or a gynecological clinic might establish policies regarding the various forms of technologically aided reproduction, clarifying for its practitioners and patients just what sorts of services it is willing to provide for what sorts of patients under what circumstances. Other policies are established at levels of varying scopes, including medical societies, health insurance groups, local and state agencies, and the federal government. At each level there arise policy questions that are essentially questions of economic planning or medical fact. But inevitably some questions of policy that involve morally charged issues arise at each level.

The range of possible roles for the government in setting policy is particularly great. The government can prohibit a practice through legislation, can discourage it—almost to the point of prohibition—through regulatory rulings, can be neutral in regard to it, can encourage it by making federal support available, or can bring it about indirectly through contracted extramural programs or directly through programs of its own. Charting the best course of action among all these options, over both clinical practices and research prospects, requires careful separation of the good arguments from the bad—an especially difficult task where moral dispute is involved.

Some of the criteria that have been espoused for the resolution of such disputes are troubling. For example, Marc Lappe, a public health official in California, has argued in regard to IVF: "The moral issue of human embryo manipulation is so great and of such importance to the course of the history of man, that nothing short of a consensus of the scientific communities involved would be needed before proceeding."[1] But given the moral pluralism that we enjoy or from which we suffer—opinion is divided on that—Lappe's view amounts to an affirmation of the *status quo ante*. When he speaks of a consensus being required before we proceed, he is speaking, perhaps unintentionally, of an absolute ban, for no consensus is possible on an issue of this sort. The absolutists on either side will be unsatisfied with any resolution but their own. Again, consider abortion. Those who advocate federally funded abortion on demand without limit of time and those who oppose abortion categorically alike maintain a distaste for the Supreme Court decision. A requirement of consensus would have us still adrift without any policy, beyond whatever happened to be in place, about abortion.

To say that the request for consensus, like the quest for certainty, is hopeless is not to say that just any policy will do. Even amidst the pluralistic currents of ethical argument, there are constraints on what we can defend morally. At the heart of these constraints are widely shared commitments to fairness, to beneficence, to a respect for persons, and to a derivative respect for the aspirations that people have. We should be guided as well as we can by the moral principles that capture, insofar as possible, the common moral ingredients that exist within our pluralistic culture. We will find that hard enough without insisting on consensus.

In the debate about IVF, Leon Kass counseled caution, urging that the members of the Ethics Advisory Board oppose lifting of a federal moratorium on IVF research until "they are persuaded that public opinion will overwhelmingly support them"[2] and claiming that "Federal support is imprudent in the face of strong public sentiment that regards such research as immoral.''[3] Kass is right that the affection and esteem in which our citizenry holds its laws and institutions are a far more important measure of our national health than is the degree of our technological progress. But I disagree with his sense of prudence in the setting of policy in morally sensitive areas. His aversion to distress, even to acute distress, on the part of a disaffected segment of the public leads him to adopt a dangerous position. For increasingly the issues that call for sensitive deliberation in the forums of public policy are issues about which opinion is strongly divided in such a way as to make overwhelming public support unlikely for any outcome. Does the public overwhelmingly support gun control, the Equal Rights Amendment, resumption of the draft, national health insurance, a balanced budget, or any particular policy on abortion? In some cases it is almost impossible to tell; in others the problem is not to find a policy that has overwhelming support, but to find a policy that all sides can tolerate, even where they all cannot admire it. To shrink from strong opposition, on some issues, is to shrink from *every* available position. On others, it is to concede the issue to a vocal, organized minority. To ask for overwhelming public support for a change in policy, moreover, may be to endorse the *status quo ante*, thereby creating strong opposition.

Policy-setting bodies therefore cannot simply be a reflection of moral consensus. Whatever the diversity of opinion about a matter, a policy is unitary. Of course, such bodies should take seriously the views of all who are concerned about the question at issue. In the case of the debate about IVF, for example, that requires a serious consideration of the values and convictions of those who strongly oppose the procedure in either clinical or research uses. But it also requires taking seriously the values of those infertile couples who so passionately look to IVF as providing their only chance to participate in the treasured institutions of parenthood, family, and lineage. And it requires crediting the concerns of those whose commitment to socially beneficial scientific pursuits is deeply felt. The policy that then results, in this case and in general, should endorse the path supported by the best reasons, not the path of least public resistance.

12

Good Doctors

WE BEGAN, in the first chapter, by considering how the behavior of physicians can fail to meet the expectations that patients and the public might reasonably impose on them. But we have also noted, along the way, that the burdens faced by physicians are severe, the problems complex, and the expectations sometimes unreasonable. In this chapter I will offer an account of what is involved in being a good doctor and some recommendations about how medical training could increase the likelihood that doctors will turn out that way. So the chapter will focus on medical education. That seems, on the face of it, a rather specialized concern, and the general reader may wonder why it is included here.

There are several reasons. First, the physician is the central player in the transactions of medical care. To the extent that we all are concerned with the quality and character of medical care—as health care professionals, patients, or citizens—we are concerned with what physicians do and how well they are prepared to face their responsibilities. We each stand to be directly touched by the effects of medical training, in various ways, at various times. Also, medical education is largely supported at public expense. Even after the substantial reductions in public support for education that have been proposed in the early 1980s, the costs of educating physicians will continue to be largely borne by public resources. Since we all are affected by the results of medical education and since we largely pay for it in the first place, it is surely appropriate to pay some attention to what it is and how well it is working. The better we all understand what is involved in being and becoming a good doctor, the easier it will be for us to be supportive of the efforts physicians make to maintain a high standard of performance.

An independent reason for attending to the training of physicians, especially to their preparation for dealing with moral issues, is that we have good reason to be concerned about the professions generally, and the medical profession can be an instructive case study for those whose concerns lie elsewhere. Whether it is a mark of increased social complexity, greater public awareness, or other causes, all our professions are having to grapple with the ethical dimensions of their professional lives. Scientists, teachers, lawyers, jurists, politicians, and others have come under the same sort of moral scrutiny that has been brought to bear more visibly on the more visible profession of medicine. To the extent that we can gain an increased understanding of what is involved in being a good doctor and what is likely to make doctors good, we will also have gained a model for the illumination of professional standards and professional training more generally. It is with this broader agenda in mind that I invite you now to consider the question, in both its senses, What makes a good doctor?

The need for reform in medical education persists because clinical medicine is based on a rapidly changing body of scientific information, because of changing social expectations in regard to health services, and because of a changing understanding of how people learn and of what it is most important for them to learn. I do not presume to offer a comprehensive view of what medical education should be or to suggest that it can ever be structured in a definitively correct way. I merely offer some suggestions about how it can be improved in some respects.

The objective of medical education is primarily the training of good physicians. It is not possible to provide an uncontroversial definition of the species. But I will emphasize those characteristics that are central to the concerns of this discussion; most of them have been addressed at least implicitly in what has gone before. I then want to consider how the goal of producing such physicians can be more successfully achieved.

Primary among the characteristics that I associate with the good physician are these: The good physician

—has and maintains a high level of technical competence, including both the knowledge and the skills appropriate to his specialty;
—is unfailingly thorough and meticulous in his approach to his specialty;
—is aware of the dependence of clinical medicine on medical research and equally aware of the experimental nature of clinical medicine;
—sees patients as persons with life stories, not merely as bodies with ailments;

—sees beyond simplistic slogans about health, nature, and life to the complexity involved in selecting goals for treatment;

—has a breadth of understanding that enables transcending the parochialism of his own specialty;

—understands his own values and motivation well enough to recognize that they can be in conflict with the patient's interests;

—is sensitive to the diversity of cultural, interpersonal, and moral considerations that can influence a patient's view of what is best, in process or outcome, in the context of medical care, and has the judgment to respect that diversity without undermining the integrity of his own moral commitments;

—has a respect for persons that shapes his interactions with patients, staff, and colleagues alike;

—has the humility to respect patient autonomy, the dedication to promote it through patient education, and the courage to override it when doing so seems justified;

—has the honesty to be truthful both with himself and with his patients about his own fallibility and that of his art; and

—has the sensitivity to recognize moral conflict where it exists, the motivation to face it where it is recognized, the understanding to consider it with intelligent reflection where it is faced, and the judgment to decide wisely following such consideration.

It is a tall order. But many physicians meet it, and more approximate to it reasonably well. The question is whether it is possible to increase the extent to which physicians on the whole are of this character.

A good physician obviously must know a great many things. Medical schools are notorious for requiring the assimilation of an enormous mass of factual material and for requiring little in the way of reflection. This is not peculiar to medical schools, of course, but is characteristic of professional training generally. As Daniel Callahan and Sissela Bok write, in their 1980 report *The Teaching of Ethics in Higher Education*:

> It is striking how few professional schools offer students an opportunity to examine the nature of their profession—its historical roots, its function in society, its sociological characteristics, and its assumptions about the political and social order. Such questions will of course arise during a professional education, but few professional schools seem to think it valuable to confront them in any systematic fashion.[1]

This phenomenon led one of my college roommates, an outrageously bright man who went on to a leading medical school, to enroll simultaneously, after one semester of medicine, in a graduate program in another discipline; this he reported doing to temper the tedium of medical education with something conceptually interesting.

It should be clear that acquiring the characteristics listed above does not, in the main, depend on the accumulation of information. Rather, they are largely dispositions to behave in certain ways—aspects of character, not merely of mind. Recall that Plato held right actions to be a matter of understanding: To know the good is to seek the good. But for Aristotle, understanding alone would not suffice: Right action flows from the will, not from the understanding alone. It was perhaps the Watergate story that most effectively brought to the public consciousness the wisdom of Aristotle's view, for the Watergate rogues were largely intelligent and highly trained professionals. As Arjay Miller (former Dean of the Stanford Business School and previously head of the Ford Motor Company) put it in a newspaper interview, "It is a problem of motivation and basic human values. There are a lot of people in jail today who have passed ethics courses."[2]

No wonder, then, that there is dispute about the possibility of increasing the extent to which physicians have these characteristics. In one view it is beyond the reach of education. One hopes the admissions process will select only people of sterling character, for with those of sterling character no moral education is needed, whereas for those who lack it, nothing can be done. A second view holds that character and moral judgment are, in fact, subject to educational influence, even though they may not be wholly a matter of cognitive understanding; it then becomes incumbent upon medical schools to provide the right kinds of educational influences. And here the sides divide again, on the matter of effective pedagogy.

Aristotle saw habituation as the only effective route to moral improvement: If you would become virtuous, act as a virtuous man does until the patterns of behavior that make him virtuous become habit with you. Then you, too, will have become a man of virtue.[3] This viewpoint is defended by many medical educators. Students learn not merely what they are taught explicitly but also what they gather from the behavior of teachers who serve as role models. A kind of imprinting goes on, apart from the transactions of textbook and classroom, that determines a student's approach to people and decisions. No other method of teaching morality or character should be employed, the argument goes, because no other method works. One must instead rely on the selection processes for students and faculty, so that the students are inclined to develop the proper habits of behavior and their faculty mentors will present exemplary standards of behavior.

This view has strengths and weaknesses. Surely much learning and patterning of behavior do result from the implicit influence on us of the people we admire. The power of the faculty member as a role model is often underestimated by teachers, perhaps because it is more comfortable to concentrate on the presentation of one's discipline than to concentrate on the presentation of oneself. But it is a failure of responsibility to rely solely on this phenomenon, for various reasons. First, faculty members are selected primarily for disciplinary expertise and are not all exemplars of the good physician. Secondly, there is the obvious problem of selecting the paragons of virtue from among the panoply of behavioral types that are available as models. If one does not yet understand what virtue is, how is one to know which behavior to emulate? For Aristotle, it is a matter of parental responsibility and of legislation. The ideal state will constrain people, through its system of laws, to act in accordance with virtue until such actions become so much a matter of habit that they persist even in the absence of constraint. Only then is virtue achieved, in Aristotle's view.[4] But it is plainly impossible to write rules of specific behavior that will habituate students of medicine to the behavior of the good physician. Nor does it suffice to tell them to model themselves after those who exemplify whatever sense they have already developed of excellence in clinical behavior. Rather, there must be an interplay between the understanding that can be achieved through thinking about questions of morality and the internalization of standards that does come from a repeated pattern of behavior. Virtue is not a purely cognitive capacity, but neither is it wholly independent of the understanding.

I once presented to a class a case that was hypothetical but based on cases that are real. At issue was the treatment of the irreversibly comatose. The patient was a young child, hopelessly ill, devoid of sentience, capable of an indeterminate life with the support of medical treatment, but threatened with a curable infection that would end the life if left untreated. This is a standard sort of class exercise in grappling with problems of medical ethics. As expected, the class debate centered on questions of the right to life, whether considerations of the quality of a life could be legitimately taken into account, why life has value, what the physician's obligations are, whether considerations of what consequences would be "for the best" should settle the matter, whether the high costs of sustaining the life had any bearing on the case, and the like. Some members of the class were uncertain about what to do, but many of them thought it was quite clear what to do. They divided, of course, into two camps—those who thought it obvious that this child's life must be preserved and those who thought that this former child, now but a vegetating relic of humanity, should be dispatched as promptly as circumstances would allow. Each group viewed the other with uncomprehending horror. We discussed the case at length, reached what common understanding we could, made as much sense as possible of the remaining conflict, and moved on.

A year later the hypothetical case came to life. A physician presented an actual case in which the circumstances of the patient were essentially the same. The discussion and debate were replayed. But then the physician arranged for us all to go into the hospital to see the patient. We discussed the case in a conference room for a while, and then the child was brought in. She was barely three, a beautiful little blond girl, sleeping deeply without concern for the tubes that linked her to the surrounding outside world. She breathed unaided, and responded to nothing. She had been in such a state for months, her condition was one of slow but inexorable decline, and no physician held out any hope for recovery. Moments before, the debate had been spirited and positions had been emphatic. Now the class was subdued, awed almost into silence by the presence of a tragedy that shredded their arguments into irrelevance, shattered their confidence, and terrified them. With tears in their eyes they stared mutely into the face of the horrible, hopeless reality. Then, slowly, they began to challenge that reality. Couldn't this be tried, or that, they wondered. But there was no escape; the medical evidence was overwhelming. And as they gradually accepted the reality of the case they had so easily discussed when it did not confront them, there was very little certainty in the air. Those who had argued for a calculated, coldly consequentialist case for withdrawing support were struck by the obvious humanity, by the beauty, by the seeming peace of the sleeping child. One student volunteered that she would never again refer to any patient as a vegetable, that although she had argued for the withdrawal of treatment, she now had no idea what was right. But another, who had argued for continued treatment, was overcome with the hopelessness that he so reluctantly came to accept. He'd always had a respect for life, he explained, but this life was so impoverished, so limited, so searingly painful for all those around it that he was no longer certain what he would do either.

At the next class meeting the discussion revealed that a number of students, including several who had offered opinions previously, were uncertain about what should be done. And among those who were able to take a side, there were several who had switched from the position they had previously taken to the one they had previously opposed; this crossing over had occurred both ways. Yet no additional information of any substantial sort had been imparted to the class in the interim—none, that is, of the sort that can be apprehended by the intellect alone. Instead, the feelings of many students had been powerfully engaged in a way that influenced their beliefs about what ought to be done. They were then challenged to consider the extent to which this impact of feelings on their judgment was legitimate. For on one account, the best decision is most likely to emerge from a dispassionate analysis based on the relevant factors that can be abstracted from a situation without regard to the emotionalism that can distort the judgment of those immediately involved in a case. Yet the feelings of the involved parties are among the relevant facts, and it is irrational not to give due weight to the nonrational factors that swirl around a tragic situation. So we discussed how the students' feelings arose, what effect those feelings had on their judgments, and whether their judgments were likely to be better or worse when they were thus influenced by an emotional response to a situation they had previously been able to discuss in a more detached way. I believe that the students gained an enhanced appreciation of the interplay of emotions and judgment; in any event, I gained an enhanced sense of the shallowness of discussion that is wholly detached from the emotional impact, and the attendant stresses, of the situation in question.

The phenomenon of detachment is central in medical practice, and it may in part explain some of the interpersonal failings that physicians often exhibit under close scrutiny. For physicians must do terrible things to people, and it may be a psychological necessity to maintain a certain degree of detachment from the patient when such things are being done. The clearest case is that of surgery; surgeons are notoriously more remote and aloof than the practitioners of other specialties and often strike their patients as being brusque, mechanical, calculating, or cold. But think of what they have to do! A surgeon who identifies sensitively with the patient on the operating table may be less effective for it, to the ultimate disadvantage of the patient. The apparent detachment of the surgeon may be a mechanism which, by defending the surgeon against the natural sentiments that could arise from and impede the doing of surgery, makes it possible to do it well. A certain amount of detachment is also a necessary consequence of the professionalization of the physician—of the development of a sense of identification with a peer group from which standards and conventions of behavior are derived over the course of a career. It is impossible to march to the beat of one's profession's drum without at least partially distancing oneself from other constituencies.

Yet this comes at a price. For he who usefully adopts the mechanisms of detachment cannot be expected to exhibit sensitive identification with the patient on passing through the operating room door. As Aristotle noted, the patterns of behavior we adopt shape the character we assume, and we become what we do. The physician who suffers along with each patient, however, will not likely be any more successful than the one for whom the patient is merely an object presenting a challenge to technical expertise. There is thus a tension between detachment and sensitivity that calls upon the physician to strike a balance between letting emotions run rampant and suppressing them to a point that dehumanizes the physician beyond the point of successful interpersonal interactions.

To learn to strike such a balance, one must experience a range of emotional responses to the highly charged situations that clinicians face— the repugnance of delivering a monstrosity, the elation of a dramatic intervention, the revulsion of mutilating surgery, the frustration of dealing with an uncooperative patient, the discomfort of reporting a death to a spouse, the anger and humiliation of botching a case, the satisfaction of doing a difficult procedure well, and all the rest. It does not suffice simply to learn in the classroom that such responses occur and can influence the way one makes decisions. But neither does it suffice simply to experience such responses along the way to becoming an independent practitioner, for it takes an understanding of the essence of good medical practice to develop the ability to strike the elusive balance. So, unsurprisingly, there are both cognitive and affective dimensions to learning to be a good physician, and there is a constant interplay between them. This has consequences for the way medical education should be structured.

Thinking about moral conflicts in medicine will not by itself prepare physicians to deal with them; the case of the comatose girl illustrates this point. Neither will feeling the impact of such cases by itself enhance the capacity to confront them wisely. Rather, what is required is a prolonged interplay of thinking about problems, facing them (in reality or through as realistic a simulation as possible), and then thinking about them again with others who can bring critical scrutiny to bear on the quality of that thought. At first the result is likely to be the kind of confusion felt by the students who saw the comatose girl. But eventually a habit of response can emerge—a pattern of thinking and feeling about cases in a reflective and informed way that strikes many balances at once: between consequentialist and nonconsequentialist values, between the patient's desires and the physician's medical knowledge, between the demands of the physician's moral integrity and those of the patient's values, between detachment from the patient and identification with the patient, and between the affective and cognitive factors that influence how one decides what to do. This pattern is a large part of what in the end is called clinical judgment, but it doesn't just happen. It is cultivated with greater or less success, depending on the qualities both of the student and of the educational experience that is provided.

If we assume that what makes a good physician is not merely factual knowledge and technical skill but is, beyond that, a kind of character and quality of judgment that comes only from reflection on the interplay of cognitive and affective learning, it follows that certain lines of approach to the improvement of medical education will be more promising than others. Let me consider a few.

There is nothing like being a patient to open the eyes of a physician to the perils and indignities associated with receiving medical care. Testimony to this effect is eloquently presented in the medical literature, in which physicians report on their own experiences as patients. Much the same message appears in conversations with physicians who have recovered from major illnesses, many of whom see themselves as better physicians because of the experience of life on the receiving end. Rarely does the experience provide them with technical data or other factual knowledge about medical care that was not previously known to them. Rather, what they gain is a sense of what it feels like to be a patient—to undergo the fears, confusions, angers, and hopes that even they face when cast in the patient's role.

This awareness of what it is like to be ill and to be treated—of the phenomenology of illness—is hard to come by in any indirect way. Descriptive lectures in medical school are perhaps better than nothing, but probably just barely. To be told that illness is boring, indeed, to know that fact and to bear it in mind in managing the treatment of a patient, still falls far short of having endured the long, empty hours waiting for the physician's brief and perhaps all-too-facile visit to a patient's room, after which the long, empty hours begin again. To be told that postoperative patients can become discouraged and depressed, as they impatiently wait for their strength to return to a level that allows the resumption of work, still falls far short of living with the irrational anxiety of fearing that one's career is over, while a glib physician, oozing confidence, uncomprehendingly says that there is nothing to worry about because these things always take a bit of time. And so on.

The pedagogical point should be obvious: A prerequisite for receipt of the medical degree should be having fallen victim to and survived a serious illness and its treatment! I have no doubt that medical care would be the better for it. But the proposal is unrealistic to the point of seeming whimsical. Yet we can approximate the benefits that would result with milder measures. Medical training incorporates a small bit of patient experience already. Students learn to draw blood samples by drawing

them from one another, and various other relatively innocuous procedures
are learned this way. The students are sometimes provided with material
that is descriptive of patients' experiences, they spend some time talking
with patients or hearing them talk during rounds, and some students will
inevitably have been patients at one time or another. Still, many students
reach the end of their formal training without having so much as spent
a day in a hospital bed.

Why not require that each student spend a forty-eight-hour period in
a hospital ward, in a bed, playing a patient role as a participant-observer
of the full hospital day in the life of an inpatient? This could be done
late in the clinical years and scheduled on the basis of availability of
beds. Since it is hard to predict when vacant beds will be available in a
teaching hospital, or in what wards, the students would receive their
hospitalization assignments on short notice. They would be unable to tell
before the last moment where they would be placed, or when, and the
assignment would in all likelihood be disruptive of their otherwise busily
scheduled lives. So much the better; so much the more valid the experience. (The incremental cost to the hospital of filling otherwise empty
beds would *not* be a serious barrier.)

Additional appreciation of the phenomenology of illness can be gained
through the judicious use of films or videotapes, and medical schools
have developed some fine materials of this sort. One of the best tells the
story of, shows an interview with, and shows the treatment of a man who
was badly burned, blinded, and crippled in a gas leak explosion. The
man pleads to be allowed to die; he asks that treatment be terminated,
and he presents an articulate and reasoned defense of his position. He
even seeks legal redress, but to no avail; the forces of medical intervention
press on inexorably, and his treatment continues. The film provokes lively
debate about the right to refuse treatment, the value of life, and related
issues. But that is not the point here. Rather, it is the impact that such
a film can have. It captures the attention of the viewer, who becomes
drawn into it, wholly absorbed in it, and often deeply affected by it. It
can prompt nausea, rage, and tears; viewers tend to identify with the
patient, to begin in a limited way to feel his frustration and despair, to
share in his experience. The film has this capacity because in addition
to being a documentary, it is good drama—despite its reality, it commands
belief like a work of art.[5]

What gives the film its impact is its quality as art, rather than its literal
veracity. This suggests a way to enhance the physician's understanding
of the patient's perspective through simulated experience. For there is a
rich heritage of literature that illuminates the phenomenology of illness

as nothing else can short of illness itself. Yet it is rare indeed for a medical school to provide for any significant exposure to such material. One reform that would improve medical education is precisely the incorporation of the literary perspective on illness and treatment, despite its apparent remove from the day-to-day practicalities of clinical treatment or laboratory research.

Consider this passage on reactions to illness, from Hicks's *Patient Care Techniques*. (Note that this text is primarily for allied health workers; one searches in vain for any discussion of the patient's reaction to illness in such classical medical texts as *Price's Textbook of the Practice of Medicine*,[6] *Conybeare's Textbook of Medicine*,[7] or the massive fifteenth edition of the *Cecil Textbook of Medicine*.[8]

It is generally accepted that illness poses a threat to which persons respond with behavior like that associated with mourning. The process of mourning can be divided into four sequential phases: denial, anger, grief-depression, and acceptance. . . . It is often difficult to determine the difference between the normal range of behaviors in the phases of mourning and those behaviors which might indicate a pathological response that requires professional help. Careful attention should be given to a patient's behavior so that expert assistance can be sought to maintain mental health. . . .

Denial is described as a defensive behavior unconsciously used by a person to cope with thoughts and feelings that he is unable to face consciously. The denial phase is considered a necessary reaction to give the patient time to absorb the emotional shock of illness and to mobilize the constructive behavior needed to cope with the condition. This is especially true in critical illness or severe disability.

In working with patients during this phase it is important to give emotional support by showing concern for them and acceptance of them as persons. . . .

Anger or hostility is a sign that the patient can no longer completely deny his condition. This state is frequently one of the most difficult with which families and health care personnel must deal. The patient may direct his anger in many directions, such as toward those who are caring for him, toward the institution, and toward the family. He may become demanding and make frequent, and sometimes conflicting, requests.

When caring for angry patients, it is helpful to try to understand the reason for their anger. Illness interrupts a person's life—the plans for the future. The individual is afraid. . . .

Grief-depression is the normal manifestation of a recognized loss. It is part of an increased awareness by the patient of the reality of his condition. He may be quiet and withdrawn, or may give the appearance of sadness. He may cry or may talk about past experiences when he was able to function more ably.[9]

These observations are reasonable and important. But compare the impact of Solzhenitsyn's description of Pavel Nikolayevich's (Rusanov's) first day of hospitalization, in *The Cancer Ward*:

> He needed support, but instead he was being pushed down into a pit. In a matter of hours he had as good as lost all his personal status, reputation and plans for the future—and had turned into one hundred and fifty-four pounds of hot, white flesh that did not know what tomorrow would bring. . . .
>
> The lump of his tumor was pressing his head to one side, made it difficult for him to turn over, and was increasing in size every hour. Only here the doctors did not count the hours. All the time from lunch to supper no one had examined Rusanov and he had had no treatment. And it was with this very bait that Dr. Dontsova had lured him here—immediate treatment. Well, in that case she must be a thoroughly irresponsible and criminally negligent woman. Rusanov had trusted her, and had lost valuable time in this cramped, musty, dirty ward when he might have been telephoning and flying to Moscow.
>
> Resentment at the delay and the realization of having made a mistake, on top of the misery of his tumor, so stabbed at Pavel Nikolayevich's heart that he could not bear anything from the noise of dishes scraped by spoons, to the iron bedsteads, the rough blankets, the walls, the lights, the people. He felt that he was in a trap, and that until the next morning any decisive step was impossible.
>
> Deeply miserable, he lay there covering his eyes from the light and from the whole scene with the towel he had brought from home.[10]

Or consider his account of the psychological impact of hospital dress:

> It was the shabby gray dressing gowns of rough cotton, so untidy-looking even when perfectly clean, as well as the fact that they were about to undergo surgery, that set these women apart, deprived them of their womanliness and their feminine charm. The dressing gowns had no cut whatever. They were all enormous, so that any woman, however fat, could easily wrap one around her. The drooping sleeves looked like wide, shapeless smokestacks. The men's pink and white striped jackets were much neater, but the women were never issued dresses, only those dressing gowns without buttons or buttonholes. Some of them shortened the dressing gowns, others lengthened them. They all had the same way of tightening the cotton belt to hide their nightdresses and of holding the flaps across their breasts. No woman suffering from disease and in such a drab dressing gown had a chance of gladdening anyone's eye, and they all knew it.[11]

A sympathetic understanding of the patient's perspective is necessary for the good doctor, but not sufficient. Some address to the moral dimensions of medical practice is needed as well. But what sort? There are basically four positions. The first is that there is no point to a formal consideration of ethical issues. This view can result from the belief that the diversity and confusion in ethical argumentation make complete moral skepticism the only reasonable position, so that there is nothing to discuss. I have argued that this is overly pessimistic and that enough light can be shed by a systematic inquiry into matters of morality to make the undertaking worthwhile. Opposition also arises from the belief that the behavior of physicians depends on the moral outlook they have established prior to their medical training. This, too, I see as overly pessimistic; given an initial disposition on the part of the student to take matters of morality seriously, the quality of moral judgment can be enhanced by a systematic and guided exploration of the issues.

Three remaining positions hold that the consideration of ethics should take place early, late, and throughout the curriculum. As Callahan and Bok report:

> A common problem in professional schools is whether it is better, comparatively, to introduce ethics at the beginning of a professional education, or to wait until the end. The main argument for introducing it at the beginning is to alert students to the ethical problems they will encounter in other courses, and to serve notice of the importance of ethical concerns. The argument for putting it at the end of a professional education is that, by then, students will better understand the nature of their profession and its problems, and thus be in a stronger position to appreciate the moral dilemmas—something not always possible when students, at the very beginning, have yet to really discover the nature of the professional problems themselves. . . .
>
> A frequent comment, at both the undergraduate and especially the professional school level, is that ethics ought not to be taught in a specific course at all, but should be built into all other courses in the curriculum.[12]

Providing formal consideration of ethical issues at the start of professional training is the inoculation method. Give them a good dose at the outset, and they will be immune from moral crisis thereafter! The odd booster shot may be needed from time to time, but basic protection should be provided.

This method is unlikely to succeed. The initial dose is often small and dilute—a few guest lectures in the first-year program, a series of lunch-hour discussions, or something of the kind. More important, there is a mismatch between the methods and the goals. For there are two distinct stages of ethical sophistication often conflated. One is the heightening of moral sensitivity—making the physician aware of value assumptions, value conflicts, and perhaps different theoretical accounts of the nature and origin of values. This much may well be accomplished in a single course. But the other objective is the more crucial, and that is to go beyond a heightened awareness of ethical issues to an enhanced capacity to exercise ethical judgment. And this requires the internalization of a habit of mind that can come only through prolonged and reflective grappling with the issues. Even a large and potent single dose cannot accomplish that.

For the same reason, the single dose will fail when administered at the end of a professional program. Further, such late administration lets pass the opportunity to provide an enriched perspective for viewing the experiences to be encountered throughout a medical school career. So it may seem that the method of building ethical consideration into all the courses—what has come to be known as the pervasive method—is the method of choice. But it is even less satisfactory than the others.

What is everyone's responsibility too easily becomes no one's, and the time devoted to ethical issues in the context of other pursuits is likely to be insignificant. Worse, what consideration does occur is likely to be untutored, providing the form without the substance. One cannot expect the entire faculty of a medical school to be competent in the analysis of ethical issues—any more than one should expect them all to be competent in, say, anesthesiology. But whereas no one without qualifications in anesthesiology would consider trying to teach it, anyone can conduct a meandering discussion of some moral dilemma or other or can ruminate aloud about ethical conflicts faced and conquered. As likely as not, the result will be, at best, to increase the student's awareness of the reality of moral conflict and, at worst, to give the consideration of ethical issues a bad name.

I favor the intermittent method. Students should be sensitized to the reality and importance of ethical issues as early as possible in their medical training. And surely at the end, before they go on to residencies, there should be another systematic exploration of ethical issues, linked to the clinical experiences they will have confronted. Along the way there should be some thread of continuity—structuring and guiding the reflections that the students bring to bear on ethical matters. For the point is not to provide information, but to cultivate habits of mind and attitude. Only if the students' exposure to ethical reflection is a continuing presence in their consciousness will this result be achieved.

The details are where such proposals come to grief because of battles about who has to give up what to transform them from noble plans into operating programs. A medical school would have to go to some lengths to make such a program a reality, but some have already done it, thereby demonstrating their collective concern with the humanistic dimensions of medical practice.

Every discussion of curriculum reform comes rapidly to dispute about whether new programs should be required. Many medical schools offer courses in medical ethics and related areas as electives to interested students. However, they play little role in increasing the likelihood that the school will produce good physicians. For the students who elect them tend to be those who need them least. The chap who is most likely to become a cold medical technician will give such courses wide berth.

In a recent BBC series on the British public schools one headmaster put his position well. "Any lad worth 'is salt," he said, "will find the easy path. That's why they must be coerced into valuable experience." The point has broad applicability, for higher education generally has suffered a crisis of confidence and a failure of responsibility in the planning of educational programs. In the tumultuous period from 1964 through the mid-1970s, many long-overdue educational reforms were adopted at colleges and universities, but some excesses were embraced along the way. One of them was an overready acceptance of the notion that students know enough to determine not only what general course of studies they wish to pursue but what the fine structure of that pursuit should be. They do not. The faculty has no infallible insight into such matters, but it does have a broader base of judgment and a responsibility to exercise it. On the basis of that responsibility, medical schools should require a sustained consideration of the moral issues in clinical practice.

Increasingly, matters of medical practice become entangled with matters of public policy. Whenever there are issues to decide about such matters as expansion of hospital beds, the financing of medical care, or the establishment of environmental or industrial safety standards, physicians are called upon in the deliberation. Although their role may in principle be thought of as value-free, providing just the relevant technical facts, it is not possible in reality to separate the issues as sharply as that. The physician as a citizen is called upon to exercise judgment in hearings, at civic meetings, on committees, and at the ballot box, on matters that pertain to medicine and health. Yet there is typically nothing in the training of a physician to provide for an informed sense of social responsibility where such matters are concerned. This, too, needs redress in the curriculum.

I have argued against the position that the morality of medical students is wholly determined by the selections of the admissions committee. I believe that students who have the moral capacity and inclination to become good physicians are far more likely to do so if they are exposed to the kinds of influences I have been describing. Of course, some students will become good physicians, as many have before them, independently of the content of their training. And others will be interpersonal thugs no matter what they are exposed to in or after medical school. But that is no argument against reforms—no more than it is an argument against driving safely that doing so only modifies the likelihood of survival.

The extent to which students benefit from such programs along the way to becoming good doctors will depend to a great degree on who they are at the outset. So, although I reject the view that admissions decisions wholly determine the moral character of the class, I want to focus now on the importance of such decisions. There is probably no greater influence on the products of any educational institution than the raw material on which it exercises its influence—the students chosen for admission. Much of their ultimate character is already shaped, and they constitute one of the primary influences on one another. Present circumstances make medical school admissions highly competitive, and admissions decisions are often made on the basis of marginal considerations. There is a substantial literature concerning admissions policies, and medical sociologists strive to understand what sorts of policies have what sorts of results. My views on the matter are not offered as the results of any study, but rather as suggestions for consideration.

Some years ago I was privy to admissions deliberations at a prestigious medical school. There were more than 5,000 applications for just over 100 seats. Most of the applications were from very good students, and perhaps the top ten percent—500 or so—were indistinguishably excellent. There were even 200 applicants who already held the Ph.D. In a situation like that, an admissions committee can be very fussy. In the scramble to gain admission, the premedical student will do whatever there is a hint that admissions committees look on with favor. So if it were known that a particular school needed a new kettle-drum player for its anatomy lab band, drum sales would boom near college campuses across the land. And if an admissions committee rather favored fans of surrealistic art, campus bookstores would be stripped overnight of posters by Magritte. Because of this immense power, admissions policies must be fashioned and promulgated with great care.

Typically a candidate must have taken courses in mathematics, biology, and chemistry. But there is no requirement to have specialized in such subjects. Rather, the student may have taken a degree in linguistics, art history, philosophy, or anything else, so long as the premedical requirements are met. Yet most premedical students do major in biological or natural sciences largely because of the belief that doing so will enhance their prospects for admission. Further, they show no particular propensity to study such areas as abnormal psychology, moral philosophy, or sociology of the family, which have potential bearing on the practice of medicine. The quest for the perfect grade dominates all decisions, and the quest for breadth of learning takes a back seat.

A handful of medical schools could modify this pattern by explicitly favoring, among those with superb records in the premedical requirements, students who demonstrate an active concern with the humanistic dimensions of health care, manifested in the sustained pursuit of programs in the humanities or social sciences or in other ways. Such students do gain admission to medical school now, but increasing their number—a transformation that could be accomplished in short order—could substantially alter the intellectual climate within medical education and increase receptivity to the programs most likely to nurture the character traits that make good physicians good. No diminution of technical competence would result; selections would still be from among the technically superior. But parochialism might well diminish, and better clinical judgment could result. The experiment could be safely tried, given the strength of the admissions committees' position in the marketplace. Of course, the occasional brilliant psychopath would continue to slip through the net, but not likely any more often.

Medical schools do not have the sole responsibility for confronting issues in medical ethics. On the contrary, training in the early postgraduate years is of comparable importance, and it is gratifying to see new programs designed to help physicians learn to grapple with the moral problems they face in these early years of practice. Nor are these matters for the medical profession alone. I have argued that a good physician must develop moral sensitivity and good ethical judgment. But as I argued earlier, the moral problems in clinical practice, although they may center on what the physician does, are the proper concern of others as well. The exploration of these issues should not be limited to physicians because such issues are also the burden of the rest of us. Those who practice medicine should be good physicians, and that is too seldom the case. But good physicians should have the support of a broader community that understands the problems they face and accepts the responsibility of sharing them.

Medical science proceeds, answering old questions and replacing them with new, often harder questions, so that it becomes impossible to conceive of the enterprise's ever reaching an end. So, too, does medical ethics change and grow. Issues in medical ethics can be explored in medical training, but medical ethics cannot be taught as if it were a body of information any more than the skills of philosophical reflection can. For new problems arise to humble old conclusions, and only an appropriately reflective individual can confront them insightfully. So no amount of change in medical education or public education will solve the moral problems in medicine; at best it can merely increase the quality of thought that is brought to bear on them.

PART FOUR

Last Thoughts

13

Regulation, Reason, and Radical Conflict

IN WHAT I HAVE WRITTEN thus far, there is a noticeable strain of optimism about the prospects for resolution of disputes about what is right. I have argued that diversity of moral outlook is not a barrier to mutual respect, understanding, and cooperation, and I have rejected the positions of the more pessimistic commentators on the current moral scene. Yet I have not shown or argued that there is a way to avoid intractable moral conflict. So the message may seem mixed. I will try to clarify it in this final chapter.

I do believe that people of goodwill, reasoning together, can accomplish much in the resolution of their differences, even when those differences involve value conflict. The dialogue in chapter 8, I hope, made this position plausible. But even there no agreement was achieved on the hardest points of dispute. People can be so fundamentally at odds in their moral outlooks that agreement is unreachable. Further, in any dimension of human activity there will be instances of behavior that are self-serving, careless, or in other ways unresponsive to the needs and rights of others. Even the virtuous are rarely saintly and from time to time may falter in their resolve to act rightly.

Both the limitation of reasoned attempts to resolve conflict and the fallibility of human motivation and conscientiousness are addressed through the mechanisms of rules, guidelines, codes, and other regulatory mechanisms designed to set and maintain standards of performance. As we have seen, such devices fall short of specifying what should be done in every kind of case, so there remains an unavoidable role for individual choice and discretion. Most of the discussion in this book has centered on decisions that fall within that range of choice.

The medical profession claims to provide adequate regulation of the behavior of physicians, without scrutiny or involvement from outside the profession. It is notoriously unwavering in its opposition to the incursion of external regulatory influence into the province of medical decision-making. Many commentators on contemporary medical care believe that the mechanisms of regulation are inadequate, however, and that as a result, unjustifiable physician behavior occurs more often than it would if there were effective mechanisms of evaluation and control.

The optimism that infuses the earlier chapters thus comes under pressure both because of the existence of unresolvable conflict in values and because of wrongful behavior of the sort to which regulations are addressed.

A number of the cases I have described in this volume have sometimes been dismissed by medical readers as being morally uninteresting on the ground that they are simply examples of bad medical practice. This has not been so with deeply divisive cases like that of the lesbian requesting insemination, nor is it a common reaction to pervasive problems like those of the justifiability of abortion or of suspending efforts to sustain life. But it is a familiar reaction to cases like that in which the elderly dying woman was receiving too little pain-killing medication, that in which the young residents performed a Swan-Ganz catheterization on the dying man it could not help, and that in which Ann's physician was so insensitive to his impact on others. Discussion of such cases often gives rise to what I call the bad practice dodge.

Physicians sometimes react to these cases by saying, "Yes, some of that goes on. But that's nothing to do with medicine as a profession because that is just someone who is not practicing good medicine." Or, "When I was in training, that would never have been tolerated, and I would not allow it on my service now." Such responses reflect a lack of understanding of the relationship between the responsibility of the individual practitioner and that of the profession.

Sartre, in explaining existentialism, observes that human nature is largely a product of the actions that humans perform. Thus, it is truly a characteristic of human nature that people perform surgical procedures on one another, but only because certain individuals have chosen to do so. That we have mammalian characteristics is also a part of our nature, so our nature is not entirely of our own making. But to a large extent it is. The human species became a species that flies in machines, reads books, puts people on trial for crimes, brews beer, attends ballets, and all the rest only when individual persons first engaged in each of these types of behavior. Thus it is that each individual, in acting alone, acts for all mankind and thereby contributes to the making of human nature.

Similarly, when one physician abuses an inquiring patient or patient's relative, it becomes true that such behavior is a part of what physicians do—not typically, but at least sometimes. It becomes a part of the nature of medical practice. Each physician represents and helps define the profession in each act he or she performs.

Now recall the fervor with which the medical profession, especially through its more formally organized agencies, advocates the case for self-regulation. If monitoring the quality of medical care is legitimately claimable by the medical community as the prerogative of physicians, then no physician can explain away the wrongdoing of another physician simply by classifying that other physician as not practicing good medicine. Rather, any doctor's failings should be every doctor's concern. For the failings of that other physician are in each instance an example of the medical profession's failure to manage its own affairs.

I do not want to give the impression that medicine is uniquely guilty of the charge of inadequate management of its own professional affairs. My own profession hardly merits better grades. The greater visibility of complaints about the self-protective aspects of medicine's self-regulation may simply reflect the fact that our mistakes are less vivid and vital. They tend to be confusions in the minds of students who ought to have been taught better, rather than deaths or palpable physical injuries. But assaults on the dignity of students are no better at the hands of professors than assaults on the dignity of patients at the hands of physicians.

In the chapter on medical mistakes we saw why a certain amount of error will always be a part of medical practice. No system of monitoring or regulation can alter that fact. Other errors, illustrated by various of the cases described here, result from moral insensitivity that the good physician avoids. I have emphasized especially those aspects of medical care that depend on what the physician does, but it should be obvious that a happy outcome is most likely when the patient assumes as much responsibility as possible for the achievement of health-related goals. When the physician and patient are working together with a common understanding of the enterprise, the chances for alienation and discontent will be at a minimum. There will always be a certain amount of residual unhappiness, however. This is partly because pain, debility, and death are central features of the medical arena, and the tragic dimensions of life can always tax human patience, understanding, and reasonableness.

Unhappiness can also result, however, when a physician simply does not practice, medically or interpersonally, in a way that inspires and sustains the confidence of the patient.

The imbalance of power in the relationship between physician and patient has made it difficult for patients to express and discuss their discontents about their medical care unless their physicians encourage such open communication. The methods of monitoring and evaluating physician performance that have evolved in recent years, such as morbidity conferences in hospitals, state medical society committees, and the like, have devoted little attention to the patient as a health care consumer who may have dissatisfactions worth learning about. The impression that is given by the medical profession as a whole is that if patients have dissatisfactions with the way they are handled by their physicians, the doctors don't want to hear about it.

I regularly receive customer satisfaction surveys from the garage where my car is serviced. Even the store where I shop for clothing has written from time to time to inquire about my opinions of the service. And we in academic life routinely survey the opinions of our students about the quality of our teaching performance and the content of our courses. Yet I have never received, or met anyone who has received, any systematic inquiry from a physician into patient attitudes toward the health care they have been provided. The mechanisms of regulation that exist in regard to medical care are designed to catch gross abuses. To a limited extent they achieve this objective, aided by the ever-present threat of malpractice suits. They are not designed to reveal and deal with smaller-scale discontents, of the sort exemplified in Ann's lament. Nor is any other mechanism typically available.

What remedy is there for the patient whose treatment has been in one respect or another disappointing, demeaning, or infuriating? The patient can swallow hard and bear it, accepting the unfolding of events with unexpressed distress. This is obviously an unsatisfying choice. The patient can get a lawyer, bring suit, and rely on the mechanisms of litigation. But that is sometimes groundless even when the basis of discontent is substantial, and in any event it is often like resorting to a fire hydrant when someone complains of thirst—there is a lack of proportion between the problem and the remedy. The patient can walk away from the situation and seek medical care elsewhere. But that is often difficult, sometimes impossible, and can be doubly ineffective. It may, as in Ann's experience, yield no improvement in the patient's circumstances. Further, unless the reasons for the change are made explicit to the offending physician, it is unlikely to influence the quality of future practice favorably. Finally, the patient can complain. Only the most assertive patients will do so, however, and when they do, their complaints may fall on deaf ears or may alienate the physicians and thereby create further barriers to a good relationship between physician and patient.

We need to fashion more effective intermediate remedies, whereby patients and their families can express their discontents and can explore the course of events constructively with health care providers. The lack of structured instrumentalities by which the quality of medical care, and its relationship to treatment outcomes, can be explored and assessed is, I am convinced, damaging to the quality of medical care and to the way physicians practice medicine. And I have no doubt that it fuels the high incidence of litigation about medical care.

To be sure, good doctors, sensitive to these issues, try to remain well aware of what is going on in their patients' minds. But we are here discussing the limits to optimism, the phenomena that give rise to conflict and the need for regulation. Doctors who fall short of the ideal will more likely be responsive to patient discontents if there is a structured way to learn of them. Even good doctors, given all the pressures they must bear, could benefit from more structured ways of remaining informed about how their efforts are viewed by their patients. Organized medicine ought, it seems to me, to be much more active in the development and advocacy of such procedures than it has been. If it is genuinely committed to improving the quality of health care in America, I would expect it to become more sophisticated in that long-neglected aspect of medical care known in other enterprises as customer relations.

Even the best physician, in open and effective communication with a patient, can face unsolvable problems of conflict, however—problems which lie beyond the reach of regulation and perhaps even of reason. I do not refer to the fact that some medical problems will be unsolvable. A reasonable patient will understand that, even amidst the despair that may accompany such tragic understanding. And if the patient cannot understand it, at least the physician can recognize the discontent as caused by a failure of understanding on the part of the patient, not by a deficiency in the medical care. I refer here, instead, to cases where the values of the physician and patient are irreconcilably different, so that no common approach to the situation can be fashioned. This would be the case, for example, if a woman seeking amniocentesis for prenatal sex selection went to a physician who was unalterably opposed to nontherapeutic abortion. It is such radical conflict that I will next consider.

Where such divergent values are present, there is little prospect of physician and patient agreeing on shared objectives. The same sort of conflict can arise in various situations, including all of those in which the matter at issue involves a decision about whether to sustain, abandon, or terminate a life.

Note that such radical conflict is not a necessary consequence of a difference in values between physician and patient. In some cases a physician can recognize that a patient's values are different from his or her own and can nonetheless decide to accommodate the patient's values without compromising his or her own moral integrity. For instance, a physician might believe that pain is intrinsically bad and should be minimized, other things being equal, to the maximum possible extent. The patient may disagree, believing it a sign of moral weakness to take more medication than the minimum necessary for effective cure. The physician may find such values alien and bizarre, without feeling compelled to combat them. Rather, the physician, respectful of the patient's autonomy, may readily agree to conform to the values of that patient in treating that patient. Indeed, much of the argument in this volume has been in support of the view that the physician should understand the difference between his or her own values, on the one hand, and the patient's values, on the other, and should be guided as much as possible, in providing care, by a respect for the values of the patient.

But in other circumstances such compromise is out of the question. The needs or desires of a patient may be so fundamentally at odds with the moral commitments of the physician that there is no basis for negotiation and no room for agreement. How can one respond to such radical conflict? Let us turn briefly to one historical example.

Thomas More was born in 1478, knighted in 1521, and appointed Lord Chancellor of England in 1529. The best known of his many writings is the classic *Utopia*, still widely read. Because he refused to subscribe to the Act of Supremacy impugning the authority of the Pope and making Henry VIII the head of the English Church, he was imprisoned in the Tower of London in 1534 and beheaded in 1535. He was canonized by Pope Pius XI in 1935.

The story of Sir Thomas More exemplifies the problem of radical conflict in values. Although he and his king were close allies, in agreement over a broad range of issues, a fundamental gap in moral outlook separated them in a way that no amount of discussion or mediation could overcome. Their disagreement surpassed the limits of reasoned discourse. The king had the power, so the dispute ended with the removal of More's head.

Sir Thomas More stood his ground in the face of persuasion, argument, and threat. At the cost of his life he refused to abandon his convictions, grounded in religious belief, about what moral integrity required of him.

In his dispute with his king there was no middle ground, no room for agreement. And we admire More for his moral fortitude, just as we admire Socrates for declining an opportunity to escape from prison and thereby avoid execution when the cost of his so doing would be to violate the law.

The circumstances confronted by More put his faith to the test, just as those faced by Socrates put to the test his commitment to respect for the law. Although the life of the physician is rarely, if ever, at stake in a case of radical conflict in medical practice, the convictions of a physician can nonetheless also be put to the test by such circumstances. For the conflict at issue need not be between physician and patient; it can also be between the physician and the hospital, the medical society, the larger community, or the law. Just as there can be an antiabortion physician in conflict with a patient who seeks an abortion, there can also be a physician who believes that abortion should be a matter of choice in conflict with a law that forbids it.

Where compromise fails and values are irreconcilably opposed, one faces limited choices. Such circumstances may prompt one to reconsider one's values and perhaps to modify them. Such circumstances also offer one the opportunity to defend one's values, sometimes at a substantial price. In the case of Thomas More, the price was life itself. And there was an additional cost to the rest of us: the work he might have done had he lived longer. In medical conflicts, the costs may also be substantial, though rarely are they borne by the physician. Consider this example.

A newborn child was gravely ill, suffering from multiple birth defects and with clear evidence of substantial brain damage. The infant had been in neonatal intensive care for several weeks, was blind, and seemed to be deteriorating quickly. The parents decided that the time had come to stop trying to save the child, but the physician was totally committed to saving life at all costs. Over the parents' objections, he continued vigorous treatment, and the child survived. Several years old now, that child is profoundly retarded, incapable of speech or independent action. The parents' lives are largely absorbed by the costs and labors associated with caring for the child. They are keenly aware that their circumstances result from the physician's having imposed his values on the situation; they are also aware that it is their lives, and not the physician's, that have been impoverished as a result.

What can a physician who faces such a situation do if the physician believes that the value of life transcends all other considerations? The physician can reappraise his opposition to suspending treatment and decide that it must be tempered by enough flexibility to allow suspension in a case such as this. Indeed, he may, as a result of contemplating this case, reconsider his values to the point of losing confidence in their foundation, and restructure his values in a more fundamental and pervasive way. Or, he may conclude that though his convictions are sorely tested by the case at hand, he nonetheless will not yield in what he believes is right. Like More and Socrates, he then stands firm and pays the price. But in such a case, the price he pays is not his own life, but what he imposes on someone else who does not share his values. He thus becomes one whose values demand behavior that result in the impoverishment of the lives of others, and which will therefore be seen by many to be parochial, inhumane, and unjustified.

Socrates and More are authentic moral heros; we see their uncompromising behavior as noble and admirable, setting examples of moral integrity that can hold a message for the ages. But when the costs of an uncompromising stand are imposed on others, we may be more inclined to see such behavior as narrow-minded, inflexible, and pointlessly stubborn. In any event, there is risk associated with taking a strong moral stand, especially in the context of others who do not share it. And there can be risk associated with avoiding such a stand—risk to one's own sense of moral integrity and self-worth. One can hope that good fortune will spare one those circumstances that require such difficult decisions. But the hope is faint indeed for those in clinical practice. Where tragic choices are a part of the daily fare, and the constituency with whom one works is diverse in its values, it is only reasonable to expect that from time to time one's values will be put to the test.

Clinical medicine is hard to practice well for many reasons. It is made even harder by the increasing moral scrutiny to which practitioners are subjected, although the medical profession has historically always expressed a concern for moral integrity and for unusually high standards of behavior. Perhaps the recent increase in attention to ethical issues in medicine in part reflects the increased interpersonal distance that many patients feel as they confront medical care of a highly specialized and heavily technological sort. For it is also in many ways hard to be a patient. And the difficulty of being a patient combines with the difficulty of being a physician to increase the potential for stress and dissatisfaction in the interactions of clinical medicine.

Despite the possibility that radical conflict will lead to unresolvable dispute and perhaps to tragic outcomes, I continue to believe that for most physicians and most patients most of the time, good medical practice, morally and clinically, is possible. Mutual understanding and a willingness to explore questions of values will increase the likelihood.

The more patients understand about how hard it is to be a good doctor, and the more physicians understand about how hard it is to be a patient in the context of contemporary medicine, the greater the prospects will be for rational cooperation in a climate of mutual respect.

Notes

CHAPTER 1

1. See René Descartes, *Meditations On First Philosophy* (1641), many translations.
2. For a report on just how much and how long patients wait for physicians, see Judith A. Kasper and Marc L. Berk, *Waiting Times in Different Medical Settings: Appointment Waits and Office Waits*, DHHS Publication (PHS) 81-3296 (Hyattsville, Md.: National Center for Health Services Research, March 1981).
3. From the Preamble to the Constitution of the World Health Organization, adopted by the International Health Conference held in New York from June 19 to July 22, 1946. *Basic Documents*, 29th edition (Geneva: World Health Organization, 1979).
4. Ivan Goncharov, *Oblomov*, translated by Ann Dunnigan (New York: New American Library, 1963), pp. 104–105.

CHAPTER 2

This chapter is derived from an earlier version, entitled "Toward a Theory of Medical Fallibility," coauthored with Alasdair MacIntyre, which first appeared in *The Journal of Medicine and Philosophy* 1, no.1 (March 1976).

1. *Canterbury* v. *Spence*, No. 22099, U.S. Court of Appeals, District of Columbia Circuit, May 19, 1972. 464 *Federal Reporter* 2nd Series, 772.
2. Charles L. Bosk, *Forgive and Remember: Managing Medical Mistakes* (Chicago: University of Chicago Press, 1979).

CHAPTER 3

1. G. Robinson and A. Merav, "Informed Consent: Recall by Patients Tested Postoperatively," *Annals of Thoracic Surgery* 22 (1976), pp. 209–12.
2. John Stuart Mill, *On Liberty* (1859), many editions.
3. See, for example, Robert Nozick, *Anarchy, State, and Utopia* (New York: Basic Books, 1974), chap. 3.
4. See Plato's *Republic*, many translations.
5. Norman Cousins, *Anatomy of an Illness as Perceived by the Patient: Reflections on Healing and Regeneration* (New York: Norton, 1979).
6. Cf. Gerald Dworkin, "Paternalism," in *Morality and the Law*, edited by Richard A. Wasserstrom (Belmont, Calif.: Wadsworth, 1971), pp. 107–26.
7. For a recent discussion of this question, see Allen Buchanan, "Medical Paternalism," *Philosophy and Public Affairs* 7, no. 4 (Summer 1978), pp. 370–90; and Donald Vandeveer, "The Contractual Argument for Withholding Medical Information," *Philosophy and Public Affairs* 9, no. 2 (Winter 1980), pp.198–205.

CHAPTER 4

1. See Immanuel Kant, *Foundations of the Metaphysics of Morals* (1785 and 1786), many translations.

2. John Locke, *Of Civil Government, Second Treatise* (1689), many editions.

3. Brian Clark, *Whose Life Is It Anyway?* (Westport, Conn.: Dramatic Publishing Co., 1979).

4. Jean Paul Sartre, *Existentialism and Human Emotions*, translated by Bernard Frechtman (New York: Citadel, 1957).

CHAPTER 5

1. See Plato, *Protagoras*, many translations.

2. See Aristotle, *Nichomachean Ethics*, Book VII, many translations.

3. For discussions of this question, however, see Kurt Baier, *The Moral Point of View* (Ithaca, N.Y.: Cornell University Press, 1958); Kai Nielsen, "Why Should I Be Moral?" *Methodos* XV, no. 59–60 (1963), pp. 275–306; and Paul W. Taylor, *Principles of Ethics: An Introduction* (Belmont, Calif.: Wadsworth, 1975), among others.

4. *Nichomachean Ethics*, Book I.

5. See, for example, Jeremy Bentham, *Principles of Morals and Legislation* (1789), many editions; John Stuart Mill, *Utilitarianism* (1863), many editions; and Henry Sidgwick, *The Methods of Ethics*, 7th ed. (London, 1907). For a sophisticated contemporary version of utilitarianism, see Richard Brandt, "In Search of a Credible Form of Rule Utilitarianism," in *Morality and the Language of Conduct*, edited by Nahknikian and Castenada (Detroit: Wayne State University Press, 1953).

6. See *Foundations of the Metaphysics of Morals* (1785 and 1786), many translations; and W. D. Ross, *The Right and the Good* (Oxford: Clarendon Press, 1930).

7. Mill, *Utilitarianism*, chap. V.

8. John Rawls, *A Theory of Justice* (Cambridge: Harvard University Press, 1971).

9. Ibid., p. 60.

10. Ibid., p. 60 and p. 83.

11. Nozick, *Anarchy, State, and Utopia*.

12. Nozick, it should be noted, follows John Locke. See Locke's *Of Civil Government, Second Treatise* (1689), chap. V; and Nozick, *Anarchy, State, and Utopia*, chap. 7.

13. Aristotle, *Metaphysics*, Book Alpha, many translations.

CHAPTER 6

1. See, for example, Joseph Fletcher, *Situation Ethics: The New Morality* (Philadelphia: Westminster Press, 1966).

CHAPTER 7

1. Thomas Nagel, "The Fragmentation of Value," in his *Mortal Questions* (New York: Cambridge University Press, 1979).

2. Alasdair MacIntyre, "How Virtues Become Vices: Medicine and Social Context," in *Evaluation and Explanation in the Biomedical Sciences: Proceedings of the First Trans-disciplinary Symposium on Philosophy and Medicine*, edited by H. Tristram Englehardt, Jr., and Stuart F. Spicker (Dordrecht: D. Reidel, 1975).

3. Alasdair MacIntyre, *After Virtue* (Notre Dame: University of Notre Dame Press, 1981).

4. MacIntyre, "How Virtues Become Vices," pp. 110–11.

5. Ibid., pp. 98–99.

6. Nagel, "The Fragmentation of Value," p. 141.

7. Tom Stoppard, *Jumpers* (New York: Grove Press, 1974).

CHAPTER 8

1. Nagel, "The Fragmentation of Value," p. 135.

CHAPTER 9

An earlier version of this chapter appeared under the same title in *Medical Treatment of the Dying: Moral Issues*, edited by M. Bayles and D. High (Boston: G. K. Hall and Co., 1978).

1. B. A. O. Williams, "The Makropulas Case: Reflections on the Tedium of Immortality," in his *Problems of the Self* (New York: Cambridge University Press, 1973), p. 85.

2. Ortega y Gasset, "The Dehumanization of Art," in *A Modern Book of Esthetics*, 3rd ed., edited by M. Rader (New York: Holt, Rinehart and Winston, 1960), p. 419.

3. Leo Tolstoy, *The Death of Ivan Ilych* (1886), many translations.

4. Thomas Mann, *The Magic Mountain* (1924), several translations.

5. See, for example, the bibliography in D. Hendin, *Death as a Fact of Life* (New York: Norton, 1973), pp. 229–41; and Sharmon Sollitto and Robert Veatch, *Bibliography of Society, Ethics and the Life Sciences* (New York: Garland, 1974), pp. 68–77.

6. See, for example, Elisabeth Kübler-Ross, *On Death and Dying* (New York: Macmillan, 1969); and R. Neale, "A Place to Live and a Place to Die," *The Hastings Center Report* 2, no. 2 (June 1972).

7. This case is re-enacted in *Who Should Survive?*, a twenty-four-minute film produced by the Joseph P. Kennedy, Jr., Foundation.

8. See, for example, the argument presented in *The Right to Die*, a sixty-minute documentary film produced by ABC News and distributed by Macmillan Films, Inc., Mt. Vernon, New York.

9. See, for example, J. J. Thomson, "Killing, Letting Die, and the Trolly Problem," *The Monist* 59 (1976); James Rachels, "Active and Passive Euthanasia," *New England Journal of Medicine* 292 (1975); and Jonathan Glover, *Causing Death and Saving Lives* (New York: Penguin, 1977), chap. 7.

10. See W. Rees and S. Lutkins, "Mortality of Bereavement," *British Medical Journal* (October 1967).

11. C. Whal, "The Fear of Death," *Bulletin of the Menninger Clinic* 22 (1958).

CHAPTER 10

1. Paul Ramsey, "Shall We 'Reproduce'?" *Journal of the American Medical Association* 220 (June 12, 1972), p. 1484.

2. Andre Hellegers and Richard McCormick, "Unanswered Questions on Test Tube Life," *America* (August 19, 1978), pp. 74–78.

3. Ibid., p. 77.

4. Ramsey, "Shall We 'Reproduce'?" p. 1485.

5. Paul Ramsey, "Manufacturing Our Offspring: Weighing the Risks," *The Hastings Center Report* 8, no. 5 (October 1979), p. 9.

6. See, for example, M. Klaus and J. Kennell, "Mothers Separated from Their Newborn Infants," *Pediatric Clinics of North America* 17 (1970), pp. 1015–37.

7. See, for example, P. Jenkins, "Ask No Questions," *The Guardian*, London (July 10, 1973), excerpted under the title "Teaching Chimpanzees to Communicate," in *Animal Rights and Human Obligations*, edited by T. Regan and P. Singer (Englewood Cliffs, N.J.: Prentice-Hall, 1976), pp. 85–92.

8. See, for example, B. G. Buchanan, "Scientific Theory Formulation by Computers," in *Computer Oriented Learning Processes*, edited by J. C. Simon (Leyden: Noordhoff, 1976).

9. Ramsey, "Shall We 'Reproduce'?" p. 1484.

10. Ibid.

11. Leon Kass, "Ethical Issues in Human *In Vitro* Fertilization, Embryo Culture and Research, and Embryo Transfer," in Ethics Advisory Board, DHEW, *Appendix, HEW Support of Research Involving Human* In Vitro *Fertilization and Embryo Transfer* (Washington, D.C.: U.S. Government Printing Office, 1979), pp. 6–8, emphases in original.

12. Leon Kass, "Babies by Means of *In Vitro* Fertilization: Unethical Experiments on the Unborn?" *New England Journal of Medicine* 285 (November 18, 1971), p. 1177.

13. Ramsey, "Shall We 'Reproduce'?" p. 1482.

14. R. G. Edwards, "Fertilization of Human Eggs *In Vitro*: Morals, Ethics and the Law," *Quarterly Review of Biology* 49 (1974), pp. 3–26.

15. Results from a 1978 survey jointly conducted by the Council for Philosophical Studies and the American Philosophical Association. Among these agencies were the National Endowment for the Humanities, the National Commission for the Protection of Human Subjects, a U.S. District Court, the U.S. Navy, the State Department, the Coastal Resources Center, the National Institutes of Health, the U.S. Corps of Engineers, and the Federal Trade Commission. See "Philosophers as Consultants," *Proceedings of the American Philosophical Association*, 53:5 (May 1980).

CHAPTER 11

Much of this chapter is based on "Equity, Efficiency, and the Distribution of Health Care," which was published in *Philosophic Exchange* 2, no. 5 (Summer 1979). The paper was originally prepared for the Conference on Ethics and Cost Containment held in October 1978, under the sponsorship of the Health Policy Research Group of the Hastings Center with the support of the National Center for Health Services Research, Grant 1R13HS03035-01.

1. Marc Lappe, "Risk-Taking for the Unborn," *The Hastings Center Report* 2, no. 1 (February 1972), p. 3.

2. Kass, "Ethical Issues in Human *In Vitro* Fertilization, Embryo Culture and Research, and Embryo Transfer," p. 29.

3. Ibid., pp. 31–32.

CHAPTER 12

1. Daniel Callahan and Sissela Bok, *The Teaching of Ethics in Higher Education* (Hastings-on-Hudson, N.Y.: The Hastings Center, 1980), p. 37.

2. Arjay Miller, quoted in Edward B. Fiske, "Ethics Courses Now Attracting More U.S. College Students," *The New York Times* (February 20, 1978).

3. Aristotle, *Nichomachean Ethics*, Book II, many translations.

4. Ibid.

5. The videotape "Please Let Me Die" was developed by Dr. Robert White of the University of Texas Medical Branch at Galveston (1974).

6. Ronald B. Scott, ed. *Price's Textbook of the Practice of Medicine* (New York: Oxford University Press, 1978).

7. W. N. Mann, *Conybeare's Textbook of Medicine*, 16th ed. (New York: Churchill, 1975).

8. Paul B. Berson et al., *Cecil Textbook of Medicine*, 2 vols., 15th ed. (Philadelphia: Saunders, 1979).

9. Dorothy J. Hicks, *Patient Care Techniques* (Indianapolis: Bobbs-Merrill, 1975), pp. 12–13.

10. Alexander Solzhenitsyn, *The Cancer Ward*, translated by Nicholas Bethell and David Berg (New York: Farrar, Straus and Giroux, Inc., 1969), pp. 11, 15.

11. Ibid., p. 42.

12. Callahan and Bok, *The Teaching of Ethics in Higher Education*, p. 74.

For Further Reading

FOR THOSE who wish to read more about ethical dilemmas in modern medicine, there is a large literature of recent work. Among the many periodicals in this area, *The Hastings Center Report* is probably the most widely read; it is available from the Hastings Center (Hastings-on-Hudson, New York 10706). Several recent anthologies each provides an overview of a variety of related problems. Examples include *Contemporary Issues in Bioethics,* 2nd edition, ed. T. Beauchamp and L. Walters (Dickenson, 1982); *Biomedical Ethics,* ed. T. Mappes and J. Zembaty (McGraw-Hill, 1981); *Intervention and Reflection,* ed. R. Munson (Wadsworth, 1979); and *Moral Problems in Medicine,* 2nd edition, ed. S. Gorovitz, et al. (Prentice-Hall, 1983). A provocative collection of cases is included in Robert M. Veatch's *Case Studies in Medical Ethics* (Harvard University Press, 1977). Issues in medical ethics as considered from a Catholic point of view are well explored in Richard McCormick's *How Brave a New World?* (Doubleday, 1981).

Prentice-Hall publishes a series in philosophy of medicine, including Ruth Macklin's *Man, Mind and Morality: The Ethics of Behavior Control* (1981); M. P. Battin's *Suicide: The Ethical Issues* (1982); Andrew Jameton's *Nursing Practice: The Ethical Issues* (1984); and Michael Bayles's *Reproductive Ethics* (1984).

More general explorations appear in *Principles of Biomedical Ethics,* 2nd edition, by Tom Beauchamp and James Childress (Oxford, 1983); in Michael Bayles's *Professional Ethics* (Wadsworth, 1982); and in Alan Goldman's *The Moral Foundations of Professional Ethics* (Roman and Littlefield, 1980).

Many volumes explore specific topics in detail; a few examples are Jonathan Glover's *Causing Death and Saving Lives* (Penguin, 1977); Bonnie Steinbock's *Killing and Letting Die* (Prentice-Hall, 1980); Joel Feinberg's collection on *The Problem of Abortion,* 2nd edition (Wadsworth, 1984); John Ladd's *Ethical Issues Relating to Life and Death* (Oxford, 1979); *Ethics in Nursing* by Martin Benjamin and Joy Curtis (Oxford, 1981); and *Taking Sides: Clashing Views on Controversial Bio-ethical Issues,* ed. Carol Levine (Dushkin, 1984). Finally, there are many volumes of reports by the "President's Commission"; see especially *Summing Up: Final Report on Studies of the Ethical and Legal Problems in Medicine and Biomedical and Behavioral Research,* President's Commission for the Study of Ethical Problems in Medicine and Biomedical and Behavioral Research (U.S. Government Printing Office, 1983).

The best source of current information about the literature is the section "In the Literature," published in each issue of *The Hastings Center Report.*

Index

230 INDEX

Mill, John Stuart. *See also* Utilitarian arguments
moral philosophy, 83, 87
paternalism view, 42
theory of justice, 88–89, 183–84
Miller, Arjay, 194
Modeling, medical students, 195
Moral certainty, 120
Moral costs, 48–49
Moral education, 194–96
Moral obligations. *See* Obligation
Moral philosophy
major traditions, 83–95
and medical decisions, 75–76
and moral conflicts, 113, 119–20
More, Sir Thomas, 216–18

Nagel, Thomas, 116, 123, 147
Narcotic drugs, 62
National health service, 132–40
Natural science, 26–27
Naturalness, 171–72
Need, and transplants, 185
Newborns, 21
Nietzsche, Friedrich W., 88
Nozick, Robert, 91–95, 110, 135

Obligation
to one's own health, 56–60
physicians, 132–40
to prolong life, 70–71
and utilitarian philosophy, 107
Oblomov, 13–14
Organ banks, 186

Passive euthanasia, 160
Paternalism, and informed consent, 37–38, 42
Patient autonomy, 34–54
Patient Care Techniques, 201
Patient education, 20
Patient interests, 65–66
Patient-physician communication. *See* Physician-patient communication
Patient role, 199–202
Patient's perspective, 200–3
Patients' rights
in American democratic system, 35–36

and communication, 19–21
and informed consent, 34–54
Penal system analogy, 5
Perfectionism, 88
Personhood, 166, 172–74
Phenomenology of illness, 200–01
Philosopher kings, 43
Philosophy. *See* Moral philosophy
Physician-patient communication
and informed consent, 19–20, 38–45, 53
and medical care discontent, 33, 214–15
Physicians
career choice, 98–99
competence of, standards, 192–93
dying person relationship, 158–60
education, 191–208
errors of, liability, 29–33
as Gods, 6, 67
informed consent questions, 51–52
province of, 10–17
self-regulation, 211–14
social obligation, 132–40
and terminally ill, morals, 16–18
timeliness, and power, 8
title of, effect, 7–8
values of, medical decisions, 98–111
values of, and patient interests, 66–67
Plato, 43, 76, 85, 88
Playing God, 6
"Please Let Me Die," 200, 224
Pluralism, and public policy, 189
Power, and physicians, 7–8, 53
Precedent, and moral decisions, 118
Prescriptions, 141
Price's Textbook of the Practice of Medicine, 201
Primrose path argument, 167–68
Principle of Autonomy, 36–37, 42
Principle of Beneficence, 36–37, 42
Principle of Liberty, 90
Private practice, 132–40
Professionalization, 9
Professors, and physicians, 66
Prognosis, and treatment options, 45
Prolongation of life, 16–17, 118, 124–25, 195–97, 217–18